DON LEMMON'S Exercise & Nutrition:
The TRUTH BOOK

Written and Cop
by Donald

"Kiss your digestive 'dis'-or

Today's Date Is:
____ / ____ / ____ (month/day/year)

My Goals Will Be Reached On:
____ / ____ / ____ (month/day/year)

IN CASE OF LOSS PLEASE NOTIFY:

Name:
Street Address:
City, State/Province, Postal Code:
Country:
E-mail Address:
Signature:

Don Lemmon's
FREE Online News Magazine:
www.UncensoredEntertainment.com

For Program Questions Contact:
Don@DonLemmonProductions.com

ISBN: 0-9713602-0-0 Printed, published and bound in Canada

Cover Design: Jason Gateman of ThinkBigDesigns.com

Welcome to the only Internationally recognized fitness program
where the author himself will actually answer your email!

HAVE FUN WITH THIS COMPLETELY UNEDITED BOOK!

~ THE PRINTING HISTORY OF THIS FINE BOOK ~

1st Printing - Burbank, California June 1992
2nd Printing - Boardman, Ohio September 1996
3rd Printing - Boardman, Ohio May 1997
4th Printing - Boardman, Ohio November 1997
5th Printing - Boardman, Ohio February 1998
6th Printing - Warren, Ohio September 1998
7th Printing - Warren, Ohio December 1998
8th Printing - Warren, Ohio May 1999
9th Printing - Lancaster, California July 1999
10th Printing - Los Angeles, California February 2000
11th Printing - Las Vegas, Nevada June 2000
12th Printing - Las Vegas, Nevada November 2000
13th Printing - Las Vegas, Nevada April 2001
14th Printing - North Hollywood, California August 2001
15th Printing - Toronto, Ontario, Canada October 2001
16th Printing - Area 51, June 2002
17th Printing - Cap St Ignace, Quebec, Canada, February 2003
18th Printing - Cap St Ignace, Quebec, Canada, November 2003
19th Printing - Cap St Ignace, Quebec, Canada, July 2004

TABLE OF CONTENTS

JIBBA JABBA --- page 4
IN THE BEGINNING --- page 6
FURTHER CONSIDERATION ----------------------------------- page 13
THE QUICK START -- page 15
THE 12 FOOD GROUPS --- page 17
CALORIE COUNTING TIPS -- page 45
TAKING MEASUREMENTS THAT MATTER ------------- page 46
BODY FAT PERCENTAGES --------------------------------------- page 48
WHY YOU SHOULD EAT SIX MEALS A DAY ------------ page 53
CARB MEALS VS. PROTEIN AND FAT MEALS --------- page 59
PIECING IT ALL TOGETHER -------------------------------------- page 63
WHAT TO EAT AND WHEN -- page 74
DIET SURVIVAL ADVICE --- page 79
DETOXIFICATION -- page 87
WORKING TOWARDS SUCCESS --------------------------- page 96
FALLING OFF THE WAGON AND CHEAT DAYS ----- page 103
DIFFERENCES BETWEEN PROGRAMS ---------------- page 107
CARBOHYDRATES AS ENERGY -------------------------- page 122
ESSENTIAL VS COMMERCIAL FATS ---------------------- page 132
TAKING VITAMINS AND MINERALS ---------------------- page 145
AMINO ACIDS AND GLANDULAR THERAPY ----------- page 164
CHINESE MEDICINE AND HERBAL FORMULAS ---- page 178
PROTEIN POWDERS AND MRP'S ------------------------- page 189
DRINKING ENOUGH WATER ------------------------------- page 195
ARTIFICIAL SWEETENERS ---------------------------------- page 199
ALTERNATIVE HEALTH CARE ---------------------------- page 203
AN INTRODUCTION TO WORKING OUT --------------- page 217
THE FOUR PHASES OF WEIGHT TRAINING --------- page 240
KNOW HOW AEROBICS -------------------------------------- page 255
STRETCHING -- page 263
SELECTING A HOME GYM --------------------------------- page 268
CLOSING THOUGHTS -------------------------------------- page 276
BONUS CHAPTERS --- page 281

JIBBA JABBA

"Nothing is as efficient as ALLOWING the body to do what it does naturally. The only way to succeed is to pay attention to the natural laws of human chemistry. My objective is met by providing you with an education system that not only stimulates rapid results, but followed as outlined, should command the interest of every physician who claims to follow a preventative health care philosophy."

This book is a compilation of all other editions coming before it. Anything missing from other editions was found to be redundant but a lot of this book has been updated and improved upon. This book was also again not professionally edited because we didn't feel it needed an editor. I prefer to write like I speak, right off the top of my head. I wanted you to know what I was thinking as opposed to someone else's interpretation thereof.

I am not perfect. I am not a professional writer. Odds are you aren't a pro either. If you go into this as a supplemental educational tool, you're going to come out shining. I am a simple nutrition consultant who spent the first half of his professional career as an exercise advisor. Bear with my mistakes and grammatical errors.

The original transcript for this manual was written over a weekend and each revision was done in day's time as well. I do not know many other people that have sat down and rattled off what they knew so quickly and ended up with so much usable information as I am presenting, so please, just take things for what they are worth. Not what you think would have been your approach instead. While the book is not professionally edited, several hardheaded, grumpy old physicians who made suggestions to ensure a sound presentation have over the years, reviewed it. In other words, before you write off what I do as ridiculous, I can assure you, it is sound.

By bending, folding, tearing or marking in this book with pen or pencil, you have voided the ability to receive a refund. I worked very hard to complete this project. You paid a fee to own it and have contact with me for 30 days in doing so. Dr. Atkins, Barry Sears, Tony Little, Suzanne Somers, Richard Simmons and Bill Phillips do not offer that much. Since each purchase is registered to one and only one user each, please simply refer your friends and family to pick up a copy of their own if they want counseling too. That isn't too much to ask. Besides, we need all the additional business we can get just to support my Chihuahua's insatiable steak and chicken diet. Are these animals supposed to eat their weight in meat and not gain an ounce? Whoa.

I thank those who supported my efforts and allowing me to hide away from the World to create this product and my supplement line. I appreciate the unconditional love and support so many have given over the years. It is said a person's life is a reflection of the support they receive. I believe we are what we are and do what we do because of the decisions we make in life. May this book reflect the support I received and the decisions I have made completely.

Once you're done reading, feel free to drop me a line. Do not forget to let me know if you want to begin or continue to receive our monthly supplement club refills after your initial order. We re-ship to you every 30 days and you may cancel at anytime prior to each delivery. You may also request we ship every 5, 6 or 9 weeks if you prefer.

In regards to the supplements or this book, we know you'll enjoy, so please do...

IN THE BEGINNING...

"In many aspects, medical science in the United States is superior to every other country in the World. Yet, in terms of overall health care, freedom of choice, sophistication of many doctors, and education of the average American concerning Health, Exercise and Disease, we are lagging far behind many countries. Worse still, most of you don't even realize it." - Thomas Edison

It took me a long time to finally realize what people like Edison had been talking about. Harvey Kellogg, D.D. Palmer, Bernard Jensen, and others I emulated said one thing, and Arthur Jones, Joe Weider, Fred Hatfield others I also emulated said another. After researching a little more, they actually said a lot more of the 'same' things than I realized. Discovering this required attention to detail. So at this very moment, I want you to commit to a specific time and place free of distraction that will allow you to study this manual in equal parts daily until you've read through it all. Treat this as the same sort of commitment you would make towards getting a better grade at school. Look at it as though you are studying for an advanced degree or higher level of knowledge. That is exactly what it is.

And you are expected to start the diet today, take notes, and use what you learn as soon as you have read it. Little by little, the results will come as you make one change after another and you won't feel like everything has changed all at once on you. Once you have read the book, read it again. Take a couple weeks each to read it the first few times, then read it again once a month until you're sure you've embedded it into your psyche. Then, once a year, go back and do it again or head to the website and discover what updates we now offer. Read your own notes. Compile an idea of what works for you so that it becomes second nature.

It'll be no time at all that your bad habits are gone and the good habits have you feeling and looking like you've always dreamed. I want your devoted attention and participation. I want you to get PSYCHED! I want you to read this OUT LOUD to yourself so you retain more of the material as we proceed. You will never again be bothered with volumes of literature, irrelevant data, fads and myths to get your answers! I say to you there is no need for science fiction when it comes to results either!

Just open your mind. Take a deep breath in. Exhale it. Regulate your thoughts. Set your sights and mind on your goals. Feel them. Become them. Dedicate yourself to them. Calculate your every action from here on out. Everything you do should be based solely on heading towards success. Visualize, taste and savor that. Feel it. Success is attainable! Welcome it, give color, texture and dimension. Allow it to happen by having so much vigor that you evoke a response so strong that it practically comes to life without you! Become thankful for your every waking moment because LIFE is a gift! Reach for the limits. No longer allow yourself to be set back. Forget your mistakes. Let them go. You have wanted to do this for a long time. It's YOUR time.

This program is for the young and old alike. It does not matter what your age is. Food goes in one end and out the other but what happens at all stops in between is what makes us today and tomorrow. Being fat or skinny only comes from your choice of eating habits. So does your health. If you do not want to eat as often or as much as I recommend, at least separate your foods accordingly and you will see results.

If you want to eat processed foods, things considered as junk by most definition, instead of taking in clean, nourishing and otherwise healthy foods, of course you will not look or feel the way you desire. Stress makes you fat even if you eat right. So relax and sleep more. Worry and lack of sleep depletes us of certain nutrients that food cannot replace. Accepting that all things in life have both reason and solution.

Know nothing needs done immediately, because most things rarely can be. Do this and you will make more progress than you have ever made in the past by living one quiet step at a time. Vegetarians especially need to learn food separation. That is the foundation of this program. By learning what is a carb, a fat and a protein, you can finally succeed as a vegetarian. Just because you only eat plants does not mean that you won't benefit by either having eggs and cottage cheese or eating your high protein, low carb foods separate from your high carb starches.

If you eat on the run and buy a lot of fast food, do what I do in a pinch, stop at the grocery store simply to enjoy tofu by itself. Are you a Barry Sears fans? Is 40-30-30 Nutrition your game? You like Bill Phillips and his Body For Life routine? Well, low fat, low carb, high protein, and even Zone dieters all must learn the food separation rules. If you want to follow a low fat plan, go right ahead. It's OK. Just make sure you take your Lemmon's Oil once a day. You need the essential fatty acids.

Those of you on Atkins, Protein Power or any other low carb program can still follow those routines only as long as you are willing to modify what you're doing a bit. Low carb diets aren't bad. But how they suggest you do it is bad. Trust me, exceeding 30 carbs a day hasn't made anybody I know fat. Once you begin to follow my suggestions, you will be surprised at the end of the day to see you are in fact, either in the correct Zone for your body weight after all or that your new low carb plan ala the KNOW HOW feels much better than anything you have attempted in the past. You do not need to be a fitness star, model, bodybuilder nor athlete to lose fat and look good. I hear it all the time...

"I don't want to be a muscle bound hunk or a breast implanted hottie, I just want to feel good and lose some fat." Not many people do want to be or do those things to look better and that's the idea. Odds are your goal is like mine.

You want to be somewhere between where you are now and where the hunks and hotties are. I personally do not care what other people look like in their underwear; I only concern myself with how I feel each morning. I like the idea that I have total control over my own health and the fact that I can go to the beach anytime and feel confident about it. If you do happen to be someone who wants 'ripped' or 'shredded' then keep reading. I haven't forgotten about you!

Even children should learn food separation too so that they can avoid bad health and self esteem issues. I know kids are 'kids' or that 'teens' like to eat anything they choose… That doesn't make it right for you to let them. If your kid has acne, it isn't natural; it's due to their eating habits. And don't expect any visible progress for a while or overnight results if you weigh 400 pounds. You won't see abs for a couple hundred pounds. Sorry. Be patient. Junk foods contain artificial sweeteners and manufactured fats that alter the body's chemistry. It takes time for them to be eliminated from the system in order for results to show.

No matter the diet you want to follow, this book will make that diet work better for you. If you want to eat less carbs, then have less carbs in your diet. If you want more, then you can do that too. If you want to eat a little more low fat or even high fat, all I ask is that you follow the rules of food separation and you will still see results. However, the best results will always come by following this plan to the letter. It is up to the individual how they proceed, I merely lay the framework, but food separation applies to all diet plans.

Is this going to be as inexpensive as junk food sometimes is? Well, we all eat. Some afford more expensive foods and others cannot. But we all eat at some point during the day and even on a shoestring budget, you can get quite far on separating the baloney from the bread and replacing sodas with something cleaner from now on. By adhering to food separation, we eliminate digestive disorder.

Therefore, anyone can become healthy, fit and attractive. Bloating, pimples, headaches... It is all due to indigestion and it also goes away when you get on this program. Eliminating sugar, artificial sweeteners and lard is important on any 'diet' and doing so does not make food separation a fad nor only something for 'health' nuts. Does drinking more water than soda, juice or sweetened ice tea really sound unhealthy or like a fad? Just make the change and you will see the change.

Don Lemmon's KNOW HOW is no fad and just because you'll use this book as a guide for all your future eating habits doesn't mean you are on a diet either. Fads come and go. Diets do not work. I, and my 'food separation' program are not a fad nor going anywhere. We are here to stay. The foundation of the system, the 12 Food Groups, which you are about to learn about, will work for everyone because this is a lifestyle modification. The concept is leaps and bounds ahead of anything else you've used. It's something you can do and no one will know you're following... You're eating healthy foods because you're still having dark meat chicken, steak, pasta, cereal, etc.

Isn't it ironic though that natural foods are labeled as 'healthy' or only for health food 'nuts' because you chose not to eat donuts and pies? And to think you're made fun of for wanting to eat good food! Yeah, they laugh at you as if eating pastries and not being able to touch your toes without gasping for air makes someone 'cool'. WOW. And who said protein powders, meal replacement shakes or 'bars' are better for you than real food? Read the ingredients on those products. 'Frightening' doesn't begin to describe what they really do for you. Despite what they tell you in defense of their products, artificial sweeteners are poisons and anything you do that contradicts what we discuss will age you beyond your years.

How important is it for you to grow older gracefully? Have you seen someone at age 26 looking 40 already? 40 is not old but if you look 40 at 26 like many models I know do...

You can be certain, when you turn 60 they're not going to look '40' unless they take better care of themselves. You do that already? Oh really? Why do you look or feel so much older than you really are? Stress? Oh please! Noah was stressed and he lived to be over 900. The body can handle stress... It was meant to. It's the repetitive undue stress that you do nothing to prepare for or repair that holds you back.

IF you ALLOW it to recover from stress, IF you really take care of yourself, THEN you will NOT age so quickly... If the outside is showing that you aren't aging gracefully, neither is the inside. Do not kid yourself, we ALL grow old. Nothing on God's green Earth is more important than human health. And let's be honest, as a society we are living longer, but we're doing it in nursing homes incapable of wiping our own butts. Improvements in medicine and education may keep us alive, but at what quality? Continue living the average lifestyle and you're inviting high blood pressure, heart disease, diabetes, osteoporosis, and cancer into your life. Get up. Eat right. Get active. Going to bingo isn't active. Weight lifting is active! Bike riding is active!

Oddly enough, Americans are the best fed people on Earth and yet we are also just about the laziest and most under-nourished Nation in the World too. So come on. Studies show that after we turn 30, the body naturally loses almost a pound of muscle a year and replaces it with over a pound of fat. They say the metabolism diminishes one percent a year. Imagine working off only half your optimal metabolism. If a 120 pound woman over 40 gains just five pounds of lean muscle, drops five pounds of fat, she inadvertently increases her caloric requirements by as much as 20%. This is a good thing. The faster the metabolism, the more fat your body fights to burn as opposed to store...

All she has to do to maintain this is exercise and eat right. You can't exactly resort back to your old bad habits and expect your body to stay fit you know. And the amount of muscle mass we carry is also a good indicator of our immune system.

It also indicates the strength of our bones, and the ability to withstand stress so we had better adapt a lifelong attitude towards maintaining ourselves before it's too late. Every little bit helps. Think of the animals you've seen in a zoo. Compare them to those that run free in the wild like the ones you see on TV. Zoo animals eat processed foods. What you see them fed during the day is just for show and even if it is meat, it's not fresh meat, you can be certain of that. And since these animals do not have the room to run or a reason to (no food to catch), they do little work and exercise. They lose their muscle, strength, endurance, and LIFE SPANS. Do you find yourself visiting the doctor more often than ever before? It's not 'just' because of aging. It's because of the habits that FORCED YOU TO AGE.

It's amazing enough the direct correlation between man and wild animal. We too used to hunt our own foods but now we buy them from a store or have hot meals delivered to us prepackaged. We no longer run for our lives, look for shelter, chase our prey, and often we do not even exercise to make up for it. Nowadays we look for every way we can to relax, do nothing all day long, and make excuses all the while for the way we look and feel. Like caged animals, we have pouches under our bellies that hang. We couldn't fight to save our lives and get scared whenever someone says BOO. We are so sickly as a society that we worry we may have every single ailment that's advertised on late night TV. If we are serious about our bodies, we must make changes.

You are just as much at risk as anyone else. Especially you drug users. I spoke to a girl at the Ms. Olympia this year getting ready to compete that very night about her irregular heartbeat. It was too late that day for her to get off drugs, but it wasn't too late for her to begin becoming drug free the next day. I spoke with a bodybuilder at the Mr. USA also this year that had just urinated blood in the restroom during his steroid testing. Listen, if you have these problems now, it only gets worse. You really do not need to continue with this lifestyle.

FURTHER CONSIDERATION

If you are on a 40-30-30 Nutrition plan or the Zone Diet... You WILL NATURALLY BE in the CORRECT 'zone' for your weight at the end of each day by separating your foods accordingly. If you follow the Atkin's diet or any other low carb ketogenic plan, just make sure all of your meals are protein, fat, and fibrous green vegetable based using the 3 to 1 protein to fat ratio rule.

If you follow a 'low fat' or 'high carb' plan, make sure you keep all carb meals virtually non-fat and maintain protein meals at no more than 25% fat. This will keep things in a low fat perspective overall. Vegans, please maintain low carb protein and fat sources together, separate from high carb foods. While beans are not a protein, cottage cheese, eggs and tofu are. Oils and nuts do not go on or with starches....

If you are a teenager, you too must eat accordingly whether you are fat or not. Just because your friends eat a certain way doesn't mean it won't affect you later down the road. Know how you laugh at people who gain the Freshman 15 or the school alumni who are fat with thin hair at 30? That'll be you too because eating bad is what got them there.

What gives you gas does so because it doesn't digest properly, like burgers, fries and chips, will also not nourish you. Without nourishment, we do not grow, mature, nor age properly. For the elderly, those prescription medications you take will work better once you 'food separate' and your doctors will probably prescribe you less as we move forward. The body works best when all of its fuels are supplied and your motors are kept clean. Become efficient and you ARE efficient. Everyone is expected to exercise at least a couple times a week no matter which category they fall into. I only ask you to pick 3 exercises you know how to perform and set a schedule to do them. Don't be lazy.

Get up. Do something for yourself. Whether you are weak or strong, fast or slow, it doesn't matter. Your strength and speed is individual, just do what you can. In time, it all adds up to progress. Finally, if you 'food combine' that's great, but this isn't food combining. It's something better. This program explains why Fit For Life and Suzanne Somers have so many limitations. You see, this is the book I wish I could have had when I first took interest in nutrition and exercise.

Being misinformed and mislead obviously gets a person nowhere. It all began, in my youth, because I was frustrated and without proper guidance. I think of all the frustration that could be avoided. if a sound system was instilled in schools around the World today. But people are in their infancy of understanding how nutrition works and dieting isn't considered important I suppose.

Well folks, consider yourselves briefed. It's now time for you to get what I call my 'Know How'... After I help you, maybe you can help me, get the word spread. 'Diet' is not a dirty word. Oh! When I say 'carbs' it is the same thing as carbohydrates... Its just slang! If you have any questions, email me via the address in the front of the book. My work thrives on your enquiries.

Without you telling me what is on your mind, I cannot make it more clear for you nor for others that come after you. Whatever your reason for being here is, you're here. So please take the time today and send me a question if you have one. But do me a favor and wait until you finish the book first. Do not be afraid to email me, just simply wait to do it once you have read everything. I understand some people will have some sincere questions because they truly do not understand, but too many people email me with questions that are already in the book prior to getting to those parts. Write your questions down as they arise, list the page your question stems from.

THE QUICK START...

1) Before bed, place a glass of water by your nightstand. Take a sip whenever you wake up in the middle of the night and finish the glass as soon as you wake up in the morning. Always drink water upon awakening, then again between and after (but not before) meals, and even before bed. This first glass is the only exception.

2) When the alarm RINGS it is time to get up -NOT hit the snooze button for more rest! IMMEDIATELY after having your water begin eating! Food is your top priority. It doesn't matter if your day starts at 2 o'clock in the afternoon. Get up and eat. If you think you have no time, move your tail a little faster. Make time. Eat before you do anything else including waiting for the restroom

3) Be sure to eat again at least every three hours following this meal. Try not to let more than 2 1/2 hours go between ending and starting your feedings. Skipping a meal is ALWAYS worse than over eating. It slows your metabolism. Eat often just like a baby does and NEVER skip a feeding.

4) Alternate your meals between four protein and vegetable meals and two carbohydrate based low fat meals each day. If you are afraid to eat fat or carbs, at least separate the animal protein foods you have from all starches into different sittings. For now, all meals should be equal in calories. Never have two carbohydrate-based meals in a row.

5) Schedule meals so you finish eating 1 1/2 hour before and again 1/2 hour after exercise. Have proteins before training and carbohydrates after. This is the opposite of what you heard in the past but it works. REPEAT: Carbs are for AFTER and proteins are for BEFORE your workout sessions. Only drink water during exercise. There are no exceptions. Protein before, carbs after. Nothing else will work.

6) Exercise with weights possibly Monday, Wednesday, and Friday this week then only Monday and Thursday next week. Determine what's best for you, but these days are typical. You can select any 5 non-consecutive days every 2 weeks to workout that you like. You can do 3 sessions a week or 2 sessions. 2 are all you need and 3 isn't always better. Perform one exercise per muscle group for up to 10 total sets a session or try the 3 sets of 3 exercises routine. End each session with 12 minutes of cardio.

7) Write down everything you do. When you weight lift, log the weight you use and how many repetitions you performed. If you can lift something more than 10 reps, you need to use more weight the next time and if you can't, keep using it until 10 are possible. When you use aerobic machines, log the distance you go. Do not try for more and more time. Try for further distances in the same amount time. Huff and puff!

8) Get 8 hours of sleep. If possible, beginning prior to 11 p.m. No matter what, lay down for 8 hours a day even if it's in segments. No matter who you are, you know as well as I do that 8 hours on your back is easy enough to perform even in spurts through out the day. I pulled it off with 2 jobs, full time study and commuting.

9) Keep your body in mental, physical, emotional and spiritual alignment. Say a thankful prayer to whomever or whatever you call God daily. If you promise not to lie, steal, swear, cheat or get angry with people, then you will avoid 90% of what causes a person stress any given day.

10) Look challenge in the eye. I do. And I always walk away proud... Take this book with you to work or along on travel. When you come up with ideas, make notes and tell me about them online later. I want you to become so involved in this program it reverses, de-programs and alters every thing that you think you know. I want you to realize it is because everything you thought you knew about fitness in the past has been wrong.

THE 12 FOOD GROUPS PART ONE: PROTEIN FOODS

I think it is easier to learn a little about 12 things than it is to learn a lot about 4. The four food groups aren't put together right anyhow and I think it is time we have it simplified. I know 12 sounds confusing at first, but the foods conveniently all fall into only 12 different categories. And this is what makes it so easy. In nature, all protein sources of substantial content are virtually carb free. They are also sources of fats. I realize vegetarians aren't interested in animal foods but if you read into my theory here, you will see how easy it is to select vegan foods instead.

Eggs have a white (protein part) and a yolk (fat part), meat has muscle (protein part) and marble (fat part), etc. Carbohydrate foods tend to be low protein and devoid of fat unless the company processing them added oil or lard to the mix. This is important to understand because the body only knows how to process foods as they come in nature. By simply allowing the body the ability to recognize whether what you eat is a protein and fat, or the opposite, a low protein, nonfat carbohydrate food, miracles occur. Confused? Don't be. That's why I created the 12 Food Groups. Now all food selection is made easy. Let's begin...

You are about to discover the truth about foods and their benefits here, but you will also learn simple calorie tips so all you need to know is the approximate measures of your selections to succeed. If you are wondering how I get these caloric figures, I read labels. I discovered over time that most foods in their 'like' groups contain the same calories pound for pound, but I still suggest you read labels for a while to get to know your own selections. All foods contain proteins, carbohydrates and fats. When you read a label, remember carbohydrates and proteins both have 4 calories a gram and fat has nine. That doesn't mean carbs and proteins are equal in energy production or that fat is evil. However, while a gram of carb has 4 calories, it only burns 4 calories while digesting.

Carbohydrates almost 'melt' as opposed to burn and this is why they digest so quickly. Fat too burns it's weight in calories. However, protein, being of first importance, contains 4 calories a gram but burns almost 6 calories a gram once eaten! So protein SPEEDS your metabolism JUST by eating it! But not if you eat it with carbs! That goes against nature! Still, carbs are important too! They are simply of no use if you eat them with fats and... Protein. You need them. Proteins contain and create enzymes, rebuild tissues and the porphyrin molecules that assist hemoglobin in carrying oxygen around.

Low protein diets lead to weak hearts. Prothrombin, thrombin, fibrin and fibrinogen from proteins heal wounds and clots blood. Eat protein, prevent strokes. Lipids from proteins line our mitochondrias that create electrical energy (some say our very souls) from within. You'll think more clearly. And lipoproteins transport bad fats out of the body. You need protein to reduce cholesterol. I do not agree with the methods used to kill animals these days nor how they are raised. But this is why I am careful with the brands I use and purchase.

I am not going to say you 'must' eat meat, but I will say you must get sufficient protein. Eggs and cottage cheese is a staple in my diet although I do not eat as much meat as I did in the past... Before we continue, there is something I want to add. I am often asked whether the foods in the 12 Food Groups are either alkaline or acidic. It may seem like that is important and it is not that it isn't, but it is not nearly as significant as the other nutritional info we'll cover. Still, since you're dying to know what I am talking about, the terms alkaline and acid 'ashes' refer to what's remaining after processing a particular food. When you take food and have it dried in a lab to a point it becomes an ash, the characteristics of that ash is either acid, alkaline or neutral. Potatoes, legumes and vegetables are pretty much all alkaline foods. Grains and animal products are acidic. Fats are neutral. Some alkaline foods like legumes, melons, broccoli and tubers (potatoes) reduce the acidity of your gut and urine.

Foods like sour fruits increase it. What you eat determines if you are off or on and hot or cold. You need a balance of all things in your life. Acid foods are the body's accelerators and alkaline foods put on the brakes. If the brakes work, but the accelerator doesn't, the car won't move. If the pedal is to the floor and nothing is there to slow you down, you're headed for trouble. Understand? This is a sticky subject if you want to know the truth. For instance, some people with more acidity in their GI tracts must be given hydrochloric acid as a remedy. Others will require an alkaline bile salt instead (pruitus ani). Since the effects of these two substances are exactly the opposite of one another, it is easy to see where the necessity for a medical diagnosis fits in.

At this point, whether this program seemingly meets your standard and fits into your schedule or not is relevant. If you are going to eat at all (once, twice, three or even ten times a day), you can still make the appropriate decisions to eat right based upon these 12 Food Groups. You will learn all that matters in making sure you have balance in the 12 Food Groups. I have made things very easy to implement if you will just follow my lead. Saying that learning some new tricks are too hard, too much, or a burden and inconvenience in any way is a joke. You eat anyhow so from now on, just follow my lead and eat right when you do. That's not too much to ask. At least then you will see and feel the difference before making the blind decisions of the past that got you here to begin with.

FOOD GROUP #1 - EGGS

Attention Vegans: Eggs are not baby chickens. A rooster must fertilize the hen to make babies. This is why egg farms do not have roosters around. And since eggs are not from cows, we do not consider them part of the dairy group. Eggs supposedly contain 'the most complete source of protein available' but they are a still a little hard to digest and because of this, eggs should be not only cooked but eaten before anything else in your meal.

The only raw eggs I eat come directly from a farm. A larger whole egg (white and yolk together) contains about 6 grams of protein, 4 grams of fat and 60 calories.

The white alone has 5 grams of protein and 20 calories. The yolk contains, 1 protein gram and 4 in fat. Despite the high quality nutrients, which are essential amino acids (in the protein), lecithin and cholesterol, I recommend having only one yolk for every three or four whites that you eat. I love farm fresh egg yolks though. Because farm fresh eggs haven't been contaminated with drugs or radiated, they have their enzymes intact so eat more of them. So unless you get your eggs from a farm, get all your other fat calories from Food Groups 6 and 7. If you didn't know it until now, cholesterol free diets don't work.

You need fats like that in egg yolks. Only by EATING cholesterol regularly is the body able to control it's HDL and LDL levels. Ironically, egg yolks not only contain cholesterol themselves, but they also contain the highest natural source of cholesterol mobilizers. The supplement industry has made GAZILLIONS off these "fat burning" compounds found in eggs (although they now choose to use less effective and less expensive soy forms). The compounds are lecithin, choline and inositol and all three are found in virtually every fat burning supplement made in the past 20 years.

Here I sit telling people to eat eggs for a more natural source of these nutrients and you're refusing to eat the best tasting part? The yolks. What, are you nuts? This means DEVILED EGGS ARE NOW ACCEPTABLE! Here's a boiling tip for you to make them. Poke a pinhole in the round end. Put a TB of salt, a TB of vinegar and a cup of chicken broth in the water. Use a cooking thermometer to boil your eggs for 25 minutes at 180 degrees. DING! Done! What does an egg meal look like for me? I usually mix about a TB (tablespoon) of whole raw cream in every 8 egg whites and 2 1/2 yolks, which makes them fluffy when they're cooked.

I stir it up with sea salt and black pepper then place them covered in the fridge overnight. The next morning I scramble my eggs without needing to waste the time to crack and separate shells. Sometimes I use low fat cheese. Depending on what else you like, I also dice mushrooms, green peppers, and onions twice a week that I keep in Tupperware to put in these eggs too. I may have some tea on the side, but I do not have bread, cereal, milk or juice with my eggs.

TIPS: There is no secret to knowing which eggs contain salmonella. Make sure each dozen you buy have no cracked shells first. After that, refrigerating your eggs will prevent bad bacteria from multiplying. The only way to kill salmonella microbes is to heat them. That means no raw eggs unless they are truly farm fresh. This is especially important for people with weaker immune systems like the elderly, those with disease, pregnant women, and pets. Experts also say that "free-range" chicken eggs may be even more likely to harbor bacteria. When chickens are allowed to run around the barnyard together, they eat each other's poop and that breeds a bad egg. If you crack open an egg with blood in it, throw it away. Do not eat it.

FOOD GROUP #2 - SEAFOOD

Seafoods I like are sea bass, haddock, pollock, sashimi tuna, flounder, perch, swordfish, halibut, orange roughy, albacore tuna, salmon, lake trout and yellow fin. They are all good protein sources. Try to avoid the higher sodium ocean water types if you have hypertension. Check with your 'fish'ician if you have questions. Some fish are high in toxins. Usually the fatty ones caught near polluted waters and the like. Most seafood is typically low in fat (averaging 23 grams of protein and just 3 grams of fat per quarter -1/4- pound). The rule with low fat proteins is that they require a little added fat to digest most efficiently. Any oil from Food Groups 6 or 7 would work, but add them only AFTER cooking, not before.

Cooking destroys the good things in fat and that's what makes them poisonous to your digestive tract. Dead fats build toxins in the intestines, stress your immune system and lead to weakened lungs and allergies. Good fats do the opposite. It is crucial that you at least adhere to this ONE law of fats. Do not ever over heat them.

If you can't stand to eat fats at room temperature, or barely heated, either learn to do so or do not eat them at all. If you have been eating what you thought was good fat up until now, this is one reason why it hasn't helped yet. Sorry, fried foods are terrible for you and not just because they are breaded. Never eat anything fried and breaded. Grains, flours, fruits, potatoes, rices, and sodas have no place in a proper seafood meal. Even when we get sushi we only have fish and seaweed with soy sauce, ginger and wasabi. No rice. When we hit the sushi buffets we load up on spicy tuna hand rolls (no rice) sometimes exclusively!

FOOD GROUP #3 - LAND ANIMALS

Animal meat is good for you, and many of the flesh foods (like seafood) are low in fat which also means you will be required to add oils to them as well for better digestion. I know, I hear all the vegetarians screaming, "Dead animals?" I say "Dead plants?" The life may be gone from animal meat, but just like a plant, the nutrients remain as long as the food is fresh and wasn't left to spoil. So just as a piece of meat spoils, a vegetable spoils too. It's the same process.

Sure there are too many drugs and the killing methods used on animals these days are sometimes less than honorable, but there are WAY more pesticides and chemicals in our plants than hormones in our meats. We need the nutrients found only in meats to live. Use your own discretion in making purchases, but at least once a week, gnaw away at something formerly attached to a bone. Birds, poultry, red meat, 4 legged creatures and other common sources of animal flesh and all poultry.

Trimmed of all visible fat and skin (there is no benefit to eating the excess marbles of fat or skin, that's where many of the toxins are stored), contain per quarter (1/4) pound, almost 25 grams of protein, less than 5 grams of fat and around 135 calories on the average.

Protein exclusively from meat is not essential to this or any program if you will at least eat eggs and cheese (although one meal a day of meat never killed anyone). If you currently have ulcers, supplement with pepsin (this will assist in protein digestion until your body heals itself) and drink comfrey tea (a special herbal tea, very inexpensive) with a small amount of raw cream each morning. This combo may also assist to heal a weakened stomach lining.

Our favorite? Fresh grilled steaks or chicken with sea salt, pepper, and grilled green beans or a Caesar salad devoid of croutons. No bread, no potatoes, no wine, no carbs. We save our carbs for a separate meal.

Essentially, it is best for you to eat your proteins first. Take your chicken for example, grill it up if you want, baste it or whatever. Do anything but put sugar or breading on it. Keep carbohydrates completely away from your proteins even while seasoning. That little bit of breading the waitress says won't hurt you, will. So just season it, cook it and eat it. Next, after it's down, get some green vegetables in your belly with a little cheese or oil on them. The reason we do this is because the body releases more enzymes to break down fat than it does to break down protein. That's how the body works in nature.

Some land animal meats are higher in fat than they are in protein, but to reverse the effects of fat storage that we have all suffered, we must reduce the fat in those selections. I.E. Remove the skin, any visible marbles of fat... You need to consume just enough fat, not a lot, to inhibit those excess fat enzymes from attacking the amino acids from the protein.

I eat chicken thighs and legs trimmed and skinned more than I do breasts for this reason. That reduces the fat content quite a bit. After it's eaten, I have spinach or broccoli with butter on it. I might have a spring salad with spinach and Lemmon's Oil mixed with feta cheese. Whatever I have, it will be AFTER I have the protein.

As far as anti-biotics or any other pharmaceuticals used on cattle or chickens go, trust me when I say that YOU take more drugs than your meat did before reaching your plate. Organic meat is no different. All cattle companies use some sort of pesticide directly applied to the animals as a necessary step in ridding intestinal parasites such as blood worms and tape worms. It is illegal in the U.S. for drugs to be used in harmful doses.

FOOD GROUP #4 - ORGAN MEAT

Organ meats are another GREAT source of both protein AND fat if bought free of anti-biotics and steroids. Vegetarians, please don't stop here, you don't have to eat anything you do not want to. I have other food tips coming up that will help you through this without meats. Organs are things like tongues, hearts, tripe, brains, lungs, and whatever else from the insides of your favorite critter. Organ meats contain various nutritional co-factors that aid in our overall health that muscle tissue and vegetables do not provide.

Their calorie counts vary widely. You DEFINITELY need a calorie handbook to check out the particulars of the ones you choose. I personally use 'desiccated' (de-fatted and dehydrated) organ meats that are put into capsule form because they supply me with those nutritional co-factors other foods do not and this way I do not need to eat this stuff either. I do not enjoy the taste of some organ foods. But prepared properly... They certainly can be tasty. I really like my liver and onions. No ice tea, no soda, no fries, no carbs are to be eaten with your organ meats.

Man, a good liver with mixed peppers and onions just can't be beat. Liver is a food that is considered a blood builder and improves the appearance of your skin. Over weight people who eat liver tend to look healthier than those who do not eat it for this reason... Did you also know, historically, organ cuts used to be the most valued parts of the kill? Meat was literally tossed aside to the dogs instead! Go figure! Because I know most people will not eat organs and not many have access to pure sources, I have put together GlandularComplex.com for you.

FOOD GROUP #5 - DAIRY PRODUCTS

Dairy foods are sources of proteins, fats, and carbohydrates. After this discussion you will understand how an innocent mistake like drinking 2% milk with your cereal can turn into a major disaster. Some dairy foods are protein and fat sources, some are protein and carb sources. We are most familiar with milks, yogurts and cheeses and we will discuss milks and yogurts first. For digestive purposes, never drink milk or eat yogurts that have fat in them. They should be considered CARB foods, eaten only nonfat and separate from your meats and fats.

Always buy yogurts with no added sugar or artificial sweeteners added. Milk and yogurts are generally about 8 grams of protein and 12 to 16 carbohydrates per 8 ounces. This includes unflavored yogurts, acidophilus (a healthy, spoiled milk product that contains a lot of friendly bacteria that are good for the digestive tract), butter milk, custard, and any other dairy product high in carbs. Buy them as low fat as possible. If there is more than a gram of fat per serving, do not have it.

Follow these rules and you just might not be lactose intolerant after all. The natural sugars in milk simply cause digestive complications leading to the belief that you are lactose intolerant as a result of eating whole fat products (you're probably catching on, you can't mix fat and carbs when you eat). Even if carbs and fats are found naturally together in milk, this isn't a mistake.

The complications are caused by a mistake of man. It's pasteurization. Scientists thought pasteurization was a good thing at first because it lowered the bacteria count of raw milk. However, 48 hours later with all the acidophilus, good bacteria and enzymes gone (this is what makes milk sour), the bad bacteria is left unchallenged so it returns and skyrockets to toxic levels!

Therefore, pasteurization may not be so cool after all. All the farting, belching, intestinal cramps, GAS, constipation and other problems are avoidable if you'll make the appropriate changes. Why do they do this? Because raw milk lasts about one week and pasteurized lasts at least two. The manufacturers of these foods say 'so what' if this process kills both the good AND the bad bacteria, just as long as it allows the foods to stay on a store shelf a little longer without spoiling. This is what prevents them from needing to buy food to replace what spoiled on them and ups the odds you're buying spoiled food anyhow.

Without all the good natural things foods before being chemically altered, we end up sick and internally distressed by using pasteurized dairy products. So, unless you use raw milk, don't drink whole milk. And if you have raw milk, drink some by itself. Whatever brand you use, sip it, don't chug it and take a good 20 minutes to finish a cold glass. Yogurt. To turn milk into a yogurt, you must first sterilize the milk then plant a 'culture' in it. The culture sours the milk, which forms the yogurt. Natural soured milk is much better for this reason as the acidophilus is still intact.

However, people with chronic pains and intestinal parasites are suggested to avoid all milk products and begin eating black walnuts or pomegranates, which break the parasites down. A good meal with dairy for me would be oatmeal, blueberries and nonfat milk or a bagel with a fruit spread and nonfat yogurt. If I want cheese instead....

Dairy products that are not high in carbohydrates but are good sources of protein and fat, while remaining devoid of almost all carbs, include sour cream, real butter (NEVER margarine), natural mayonnaises and my favorite, cheese. When I say cheese, I am talking hard cheeses that break easily and aren't creamy. I like provolone, smoked Gouda, feta on Greek Salads, cheddar, mozzarella, jack, Swiss, Parmesan, Romano and such. The easiest to digest cheeses are anything crumbly. I always have a little cheese with my meats and salads. The calcium in cheese balances the phosphorus levels in meat. A little cheese can and probably should be had with meat or eggs anytime you eat them.

Most contain around 7 grams of protein, 1 or 2 carbohydrates, 8 grams of fat, and about 110 calories an ounce. I try to get low fat sources. The only difference is less fat. In regards to butter and creams, they are fats so make sure you read the labels and know how much you're having when you select them. I put cheese in my eggs, on my salads, and sometimes on steamed veggies. I never put cheese on breads or potatoes... The only reason that you might think you are lactose intolerant is because you have problems with processed cheeses that are mixed with sugars to make them creamy. Rarely do whole cheeses cause digestive disorder. I would suggest only eating cheese that crumble or breaks for the time being such as goat, feta, and bleu etc if you are certain you're currently sensitive to dairy products. I bet your sensitivity goes away in no time.

Another of my favorites: Nonfat cottage cheese with Lemmon's Oil, ginger, allspice, nutmeg and cinnamon. No fruit, no berries, no brown sugar, no carbs or bagels… It's a high protein food. So no carbs allowed other than the 2 or 3 grams found naturally in it. I add just enough oil in it for a 3 to 1 ratio of protein to fat. A cup and a half of nonfat cottage cheese has 45 grams of protein so I add a TB of oil, which is 15 grams of fat to balance things out. 15 times 3 is 45. The same goes for whey protein. Whey protein is in fact a dairy protein too.

Considering it is low fat naturally, it should be mixed with a third the amount of calories in fat grams from cream to digest properly. Yes, this is safe and will not raise your cholesterol levels.

I personally freeze my cream in ice cubes, 2 TB in each cube or so and then I add them to the whey when the time comes. In fact, there was a point in time I was using well over a quart of cream a day doing this with no ill effects.

But you see, the decision of what dairy product to eat is based upon what else you would plan to eat at that meal. For instance, cream cheese is bought fat free if you are using it on breads or bagels. This is because carb meals are meant to be fat free. But regular whole fat cream cheese goes great on meats or veggies as a dip.

Sour cream can be bought fat free for potatoes but you'll use whole fat for meats and veggies. And sorry, but it goes without saying that unless you can find an ice cream or salad dressing that is both fat free and contains no artificial sugars (no added table sugar at all either), it's off limits. Too many low fat versions of snacks and dressings are just sugar filled nightmares waiting to fatten you up.

Note. When you are down to losing those last 5 or 10 pounds, I would suggest dropping all dairy products that are not pasteurized with the exception of a little real butter with fibrous veggies at meat meals. Contact a farm near you for cream and milk if your grocer hasn't been helpful. Not all health food store employees have a clue what you're talking about cause they don't walk the walk...

If you want what we consider to be the best blend (a secret blend) of the most absolutely pure protein powder available, visit: CompleteProteinPowder.com

FOOD GROUP #6 - NUTS AND SEEDS

Nuts and seeds are regarded by vegetarians to be sources of protein and thought of by weight watchers as too fatty, but they also contain a considerable amount of carbs too, so low carb dieters shun many of these tasty treats. Who is right? Well, I call them fats because that is the predominant nutrient inside of them. There's two or three times more fat than protein but more protein than carbs, so... So, folks, they are FATS... But still, are they fattening? Only if you're eating creamy butter blended or roasted with hydrogenated oils, sugar or corn syrup as most name brands do. Plain nuts and seeds are good for you and hardly fattening. Phyto-nutrients, the powerful healing components found within plant foods that, like the ones in herbs, have regenerative properties. These factors are also found in some nuts and seeds, which stimulate you to burn fat.

Chestnuts, cashews, peanuts, almonds, pecans, macadamias, walnuts, pistachios, pine nuts, sunflower seeds, etc. are great choices. Go for the dry roasted only if you cannot purchase them in the raw. An ounce (1 oz.) of nuts/seeds or nut/seed butter contains on the average around 7 grams of protein, 7 carbs, 14 grams of fat and about 182 calories. DEFINITELY read your labels and look for coconut, cottonseed or any other oils used in the packaging.

Now, here's the deal. I take a half dozen different nuts and seeds then blend them in my peanut butter machine. When it is done, I mix in whey protein and Lemmon's Oil. From there, I have a higher protein, healthy fat spread, that I put on celery for a wonderful mid day snack. Just watch yourself. A little goes a long way. TIP: People with parasites should be sure to have black walnuts in their diet because that particular nut's enzymes inhibit parasite growth. Remember, fats do not go with starches. This means no peanut butter sandwiches unless your grocer carries that virtually nonfat peanut spread I use! Soybeans fall into this category if you look at the caloric content of soy products.

Tofu for instance has a 2 to 1 ratio of protein to fat. The carbs are pretty low. Some brands are bought fat free. I buy one carton that is fat free, then add it to some 'whole fat' brand I also like, stir fry them up with bok choy, peppers, mushrooms, etc, and love the feeling of eating clean, vegetarian food. Sometimes I have a handful of roasted soybeans (which are a little higher in fat) and wash them down with a glass of whey protein. Soy isoflavones are a hot topic these days. These 'isoflavones' are really phytoestrogens, which in turn are simply plant chemicals that mimic the estrogen found normally in humans. Plant estrogens are thought to be beneficial in controlling estrogen fluctuations during and after menopause but they also compete for the same estrogen receptors as your natural hormones which block estrogen from doing it's job. This promotes estrogen based breast tumors.

So like it or not, too much soy can throw hormones out of balance, causing thyroid issues, irregular menstrual cycles and even infertility. A serving of tofu, miso, tempeh, soymilk or soybeans have about 40 mg of isoflavones each. Soy hot dogs or cheese have lower amounts of isoflavones because of processing. Soy sauce has almost none. Most clinical studies that show a problem with excess isoflavones had subjects ingesting 300 mg or more a day. Beneficial results without complication occur using 50 to 100 mg. I personally use soy as a food but I don't exceed 100 mg a day. But we all know someone who suffers one or more rather odd or troublesome health issues. The majority of these people are women and vegetarians… Go figure. That protein powder I mentioned has a little soy in it, not a lot, but it compliments the mix…

FOOD GROUP #7 - FATS AND OILS

Listen, let's get something straight, high fat diets do not work like they say they do and this program is NOT a high fat diet. However, without fats in the diet at all, oxygen can't reach your brain.

So for those of you who are fat deficient, grab a tablespoon of Lemmon's Oil, put your thinking cap on, and let's learn a little something about that taboo nutrient you feel is so scary. For those of you who do eat fat, keep in mind, you may still be doing something wrong, keep reading.

For instance, you can't eat fats before eating protein. You should instead eat them during or after having the protein food. You also shouldn't exceed the recommended fat intake I've suggested either. If you do, the fats you eat may inhibit the secretion of the digestive juices upon the protein. This leaves them poorly broken down. And if the right amount of fat at your protein meal is not naturally contained in your protein food source, you must always add more afterwards along with some green vegetables like a salad, green beans, spinach or broccoli. The same applies to greens as the fats. They are best eaten after, not before the meal.

I realize these veggies have a little carbohydrate in them but it's a fibrous carbohydrate, not a starchy carbohydrate. Fibrous vegetables offer added benefit by delaying the potential adverse reaction of fat enzymes upon your proteins by binding with the fat. As long as you keep that 3 to 1 ratio of fat to protein I mentioned in mind when adding fat to a meal, you'll be fine. Yes, I am sure the little bit of fat in your canned tuna or chicken breast is not enough to assist digestion. Why? Since we take the skin off of our meats because that is where animals and fish store toxins, we obviously lose some fat content.

This is good, but the fat needs to be replaced. We're being smart about it and adding something healthy like real butter on the greens (salted or unsalted doesn't matter) to replace the unhealthy. Just do not cook with butter or any other oil with the exception of possibly using olive, sesame or coconut oil under medium heat at best. High heat destroys fats and turns them poisonous instead of nutritious. Technically it hydrogenates them.

Cook your food first, then pour the oil or butter on AFTER WARDS. Butter? Yes. We will NEVER use margarine on this program. One of THE BIGGEST misconceptions in the WORLD is that margarine somehow reduces cholesterol because it contains none. Butter contains natural cholesterol AND cholesterol metabolizing nutrients. Margarine does not. Margarine, like the coconut oil used in commercial baked goods, is made from hydrogenated oils, the body's silent enemy. The coconut oil I use for cooking is not the same oil as in baked goods and meal replacements. That stuff has been hydrogenated too. Ours is unprocessed… You want fats that are nourishing and build up your health, not deplete it.

What other fats do I use? I use my own oil blend, Lemmon's Oil, for the most part. 1 TB is perfect for most salads and meeting your essential needs. Treats? I use 3 TB of heavy whipping cream in my occasional Java. I look forward to my cup of 'Joe' because of that cream. By the way, I used to be a coffee-a-holic but I cut back once and my adrenal system became stressed. If you get tired after having coffee, it's time for a 'coffee' break. I feel fantastic having coffee only mid afternoons, 3 days a week, never in the mornings, nor late at night. If we do have morning coffee, it is one of those naturally caffeine free brands. De-caffienated coffees have bleaches in them.

If you are an addict, trust me, only once you wean off caffeine will you know how well the body actually works. Caffeine limits your body's ability to function properly. Until you clean yourself up, you really don't remember how energetic the body can be. Dressings! You can sparingly use fatty dressings on salads if they are eaten with proteins (eggs or meats) devoid of croutons and pasta or other carbs. By fatty, I mean a dressing that has only a couple carbohydrates in it and is mostly fat like bleu cheese, ranch, or even Caesar. If you decide to have a salad with a carbohydrate meal, use an unsweetened nonfat dressing instead. Read labels so you can stay within these parameters.

To keep from going over board, have the dressing on the side. Dip your fork in it before taking a bite of salad and you'll finally control unwitting overloading. A tablespoon serving of oil, butter or dressing generally contains almost 14 grams of fat, no carbs, no protein and 126 calories. The official Don Lemmon "Lemmon's" Oil, is a perfect blend of several different oils that contains 50% Omega 3, 20% of both Omega 6 and Omega 9 then 10% more from other essential fat sources. For more, see PerfectEFAOilBlend.com. It has a thick feel, a nourishing dark look and a fresh nutty taste.

No other blend has any comparison whatsoever to this oil and what it does for you. A tablespoon or two of Lemmon's Oil essential fatty acids a day, will be just enough to keep the doctor at bay. This stuff is awesome. It regulates your hormones, your cells, everything. The special fats we use carry oxygen to our cells too. This makes them more receptive to your other nutrients. So you need them. The body wasn't designed to live off what it makes from other food sources. While it's true the body can make Omega 3 from the fat found in soybean oil this process skips a beat in the natural biochemistry of the body.

Just like we humans may have similar bits and pieces that cannot be exchanged, we can't equally exchange blood types any better than can we get the 'same' substances from exchanging DIFFERENT food groups. All things require or sometimes do not require a more or less of a complicated process for processing so you must remain aware of each food substance you consume.

I don't want anybody to think I mean medium chain triglycerides when I say ESSENTIAL Fatty Acid because the hype behind MCT's are unfounded. You may be curious about MCT or Medium Chain Triglyceride oils. I would rather you not use extra MCT's. They are not essential fats. They are also unavailable as the effective 8-chain oils they used to be. They need to be taken in amounts too large to be financially feasible.

Using them even just before a workout for energy doesn't assist you in burning extra body fat so why bother? MCT's are simply saturated fats derived from tropical oils. Despite what you may hear, what you will find on the market these days is a single 10-chain lipid, which has no fat burning characteristics. In fact, they will only MAKE you fat, upset your stomach and deplete you of your essentials. You can't even buy MCT's in America that do what you expect of them without a prescription.

TIP: If you find at any time during the day you crave sugar, this is a signal of either you are not eating enough or that you are actually burning body fat. If you 'give in' and eat carbohydrates when you crave carbohydrates, you will shut off your fat burning mechanisms. If you start craving pizza, ice cream, pasta etc. now you know why. But you probably didn't know you can eat anything and the cravings will disappear. So be wise, have protein and fat instead from now on. If I crave sugar when I am done eating protein and fats, I know I didn't have enough fat at my meal. In fact, if I begin craving sugar at any time that tells me my blood sugar is low.

I know at that moment my body is going to begin BURNING fat but not if I eat sugar during a craving. If I do that, the fat burning shuts down. Listen to your body and you can't lose. When you are looking for essential fatty acids, I use not only my own Lemmon's Oil but also several other fat sources individually because I truly enjoy their taste. Almost daily, I have wheat germ oil, pumpkin seed butter, coconut butter, olive oil, chili oil, sesame oils and others. I only purchase them from one company, the same that creates mine. If you are interested in viewing my complete grocery list online, simply send me an email and I will direct you to it.

Keep something else in mind; the oil you buy does not need to be in glass bottles to protect it. The additional weight of glass increases the shipping rates, therefore cost of your oils. It isn't that plastic is cheaper either.

Glass bottling sounds like a good idea but do you know how long an oil would have to sit in a bottle to begin absorbing anything from it's bottle? Years.

FOOD GROUP #8 - FIBROUS GARDEN VEGETABLES

Gas.... It's all about indigestion. Gas forming organisms in your gastro-intestinal tract are only alive because of an alkaline environment. If you add a little acid, they die. This is why I eat cabbage products like Sauerkraut, which ferment in the intestines, producing lactic acid and balances the pH of the rectum. That's a good thing. So all things considered, eat your vegetables, like them or not. I have low fat sausage with my Sauerkraut... If you do not like vegetables, start with one bite this week, and two bites next week, three the following until a full serving is possible. This applies to those of you with irritable bowel too. You MUST.

Parts of all vegetables you purchase are dead. The natural enzymes that are in them have already caused many of their important parts it to visibly decay. At least 25% of the vital nutrients are missing from the freshest of our foods and it would be smart to take a supplement to replace them. Fresh or frozen, these treats are valuable sources of many things including fibrous bulk or "FIBER" which keeps everything sliding through your intestines smoothly. This is important because if the backside is clogged up, the rest of the process isn't going to function correctly either.

Fibrous vegetables do contain some carbs but these carb sources are not digested like starches. While counted in your calories, they are not significant. A pound of veggies yield around 2 or 3 grams of protein, 5 or 6 carbohydrates and about 30 calories per 4 oz. That's 100 calories or so compared to 300 or 500 calories a pound for starchy carbs like grains, potatoes or legumes.

Every body needs more fiber in their diet and green plants not only provide them but also can actually be eaten with every meal so there is no excuse to avoid them. I mean this.

Garden vegetables are usually very low in carbohydrates and calories so they fit well with anything. But at LEAST eat them with the protein and fat meals. They truly are a must to enhance digestion. Vegetables come in a variety of different vehicles, each containing different nutrient profiles although they have the same calories for the most part. They come yellow, red, green, and orange in color. There's so many and I use as 5 or 6 of them at a time in salads! I do however save the starchier vegetables for carb meals instead of having them in protein salads.

We regularly head out for salads with salmon, chicken, turkey, ham, eggs, cheddar cheese, feta cheese, bleu cheese, olives, romaine lettuce, spring greens, mushrooms... You get the picture... Vegetables contain things that assist us in the efficient use of many of the other nutrients we eat and these things actually fight disease. These beneficial plant chemicals are called 'phyto-nutrients' and 'botanical factors'. That's why pills and multi-vitamins aren't good alone and you should take supplements with meals. No matter the quality or content (of which mine are the foremost), supplements still lack what's in food to allow them to assimilate: PHYTO-NUTRIENTS.

The fibrous veggies that go with protein and fat meals are sprouts, celery, endives, collards, spinach, chard, okra, herbs, kale, leeks, mushrooms, asparagus, lettuces like bibb or watercress (not iceberg however), cabbages (green and red), onions, seaweeds, radishes, mustard greens, cucumbers... Wow. That's a lot, and just examples. I think you get the idea. You can have all of the above with starches too. You can also have roots (like carrots, squashes), rutabaga, zucchinis, beets, different escarole, artichokes, cauliflower, eggplants, and turnips with your starches.... Just not with your proteins... Why?

THE 12 FOOD GROUPS PART TWO: CARB FOODS

Because these foods ARE starches… Low calorie sources, yes, but starches nonetheless. You need the fiber to bind with even the tiniest amount of cholesterol so it can be used efficiently. Cholesterol has to be bound in order to cross the intestine lining and circulate back successfully to the liver to regulate your hormones and such. My favorite: Spinach, fried on medium heat in garlic, peppers and olive oil! Italian greens are GREAT as long as you do not add the beans to them! Some chicken marsala prepared correctly alongside those greens and I am in Heaven!

CARBOHYDRATE foods naturally come almost always 'fat free' in nature, which is obviously how the human body was designed to digest them. But read all labels, especially the ingredient lists. Carb foods can contain some evil stuff in them. A banana is a banana but pastas, instant potatoes, seasoned rices, and snack foods are all processed foods with chemicals in them. Carbs have within them nutrients that you'll never receive via fats or proteins, so you should eat them, but only the cleanest of selections are recommended.

Many vegetables contain phyto-estrogens, which can affect the body's healthy estrogen levels. Some are good; some are bad. Most vegetables heal you but some have been commercially altered and harm you. Beer contains estrogen too but what beer does to you is completely different than what vegetables do for you. While veggies aren't alcohols and all foods we eat are eventually turned into alcohols, when we drink an alcoholic beverage, it skips a natural biochemical process within all of us and that's the real problem. So, beer is out. And so are sugars. Don't have them. For one, make sure you aren't having healthy, fibrous carb sources mixed with extra (hidden) SUGARS. Juices that contain corn syrup need to be eliminated entirely from your diet. NO Gator-aid or Kool-aid is allowed. NO breading, ketchup, sauces, etc. It all adds up to be extra sugar somewhere along the line that you do not need. So, watch out.

Those of you on high protein plans, you can stick with what you learned up to this point. No sweat. But those of you not making the progress you're seeking, read on. I simply suggest you add a carbohydrate meal after each weight training session. But you don't have to. As long as you follow the 3 to 1 rule, you should get by without complication. Just realize your health depends upon these decisions.

While a 'reduced' carb diet does stimulate fat loss, a no-carb diet is NOT the ticket to success. The average person, male or female, naturally stores 100 to 300 essential grams of carbohydrates inside their bodies, depending on their size and muscularity. Where in the body? Some carbohydrate is always in the blood stream, 1/4 is in the liver and the rest is in your muscle. That's anywhere from 400 to in some cases, 1200 calories of carbs stored within us at any one time. That's technically enough to go without food for a day if necessary. But this carb supply (known as glycogen) depletes when we exercise and it needs replaced. If it isn't, our muscles are turned into sugar to save the organs from being broken down.

It is not a fat burning process that we experience when we are low on carbs. It is ketosis. The burning of ketones which come from amino acids (proteins, muscle) NOT fat... So, we at least need to replace carbs lost from exercise to preserve muscle tissue. Having a carb meal after training is a step in the right direction and 2 carb meals a day will satisfy most all of us. I am dead serious about your eating carbs separate from proteins and fats. Starches, as essential and healthy as they are, can be as bad as any other sugar if eaten with fats and proteins. That is, unless of course, it is naturally found within the protein or fat source itself like with nuts or seeds. NEVER add starches to a fat or protein source on your own. If a food contains all three macronutrients at once (carbs, fats, proteins), you can still eat it, but have it separate from any other foods. In most cases, there isn't a worry in minimal amounts, like slivered almonds on your chicken. But if you're literally pouring it on, STOP.

How do you determine what is low fat enough of a carb food? Multiply the total fat grams by 9 and divide that number by the total calories. If it isn't less than 10%, don't eat it.

FOOD GROUP #9 - BEANS AND LEGUMES

Beans are something vegetarians think are protein sources but they are not a substantial protein source. They are however a grand source of complex fibers known as fructo-oligo saccharides. These fibers contain a bulk which humans do not digest, but use it as nourishment of healthy bacteria in our bowels. Baked beans have a bad reputation for giving you gas but it is only due to the bacon and sugar you load on them, not because you ate them alone. If you eat beans regularly by themselves, gas will eventually disappear into thin air.... Without odor...

Examples of good legume selections are lima, pinto, kidney, lentil, black, chick, garbanzo, navy, cow, fava, red, butter beans, or blackeye peas... Every type of bean except string green and wax beans are complex starchy carb sources. Green and wax beans are low in carbohydrate, high in fiber and are better suited for one of the upcoming 12 Food Groups. The same goes with peas and corn. Most people consider them grains, but they fall more closely in line with the nourishment provided by legumes.

Beans (peas and corn too) contain approximately 75 calories, 4 grams of protein and 15 carbohydrates per 4 ounces (oz). How do I eat beans? I will make my own from dehydrated or I will eat frozen and I sometimes have canned but I never eat beans, which are packed or stored in sugars or corn syrups. Once I have read the labels to be sure, I will mix salsa with peas and black beans... I often make navy beans with fat free dumplings... I also love my rice and red beans with Cajun spices.... And I make a 4 bean chili that most chefs would envy... Peas, black beans and salsa or corn and peppers... All good mixes...

As long as all items from Food Groups 1 through 7 are kept away from them...

FOOD GROUP #10 - BREADS, CEREALS, AND GRAINS

Grains are high quality starchy carbohydrates that contain soluble fiber and come from the likes of brown or wild rice, flours such as, barley, millet (which is a non-gluten grain), rye, wheat, pumpernickel, oats, and bulgur which are all used to make cereals, breads, and such. Grains are really most anything that's a tan-like pasta, or pancakes but NOT beer. Remember, beer contains hops, which contain estrogen, which is something that causes fat cells to expand. Abstain from beer if you have a 'beer belly.' If it don't look good, you don't look good!

Snacks like fig newtons, muffins, cakes and others are all A-OK if they are truly made from whole grains and contain no added sugars or fats. As far as what I eat, I eat whole grains (outer bran, inner endosperm and sprouting germ all intact) and avoid processed products as much as possible. For instance, let's look at wheat. Wheat starts off as a berry. It looks like a grain of rice and is then broken down in a milling process under a roller. The germ, the bran and the carbohydrates are all separated this way. The carbohydrates inside are then pulverized into flour (eventually bleached white), but the germ (the brown part, containing the oil and vitamin E) and bran (containing the B-vitamins) are thrown aside.

What do they do with it all? Pigs are fed the germ, cows are fed the bran, and we humans are left with white useless filling. That is the problem with refined flour. The nutrients are gone and it is virtually useless. Whole grains and cereals are GREAT for you and generally contain 4 grams of protein, 20 carbohydrates, and 1 gram of fat per 100 calories or so. Many flours are merely colored to look 'whole' grain... Always read your food labels first to be certain what you are getting into checking for added fats or sugars. I cannot repeat that statement often enough.

FOOD GROUP #11 - POTATOES

Contain both starches and sugary carbohydrates. All types of potatoes or 'tubers' (including pumpkin) are rich in the very powerful healer, potassium chloride, so even if it's just once in a while, work them into your diet. Red, yellow, baking, sweet, yam, purple, Yukon... Nothing beats a baked potato topped with nonfat butter, onions and nonfat soy bacon flavored bits or a yam with cinnamon and nonfat cream! Mmmmm!

Something the size of a medium potato (3 oz.) should have around 3 grams of protein, 22 carbohydrates and 100 calories. Although they contain both starch and sugars, these are natural sugars and a healthy combo in this case. Again, the key is no ADDED sugar... One of my treats is sliced potatoes sprinkled with sea salt and baked in the oven. I dip them in no sugar added tomato sauce. During the holidays I make stuffing without added fat, mix in peas, mushrooms and bake not only a yam, but a sweet potato for one of my meals. Alright, I lied. I eat this same meal 3 or 4 times on Holidays!

My ham, turkey and prime rib (our holiday meats) are eaten with fresh broccoli dipped in garlic butter. Vegans, just so you're not left out, I also love those 'fake' turkey dinners available at most health food stores. I guess I've just admitted to eating like a horse on holidays too. The differences are that I do not mix the foods or meals incorrectly, I do not pass out after over eating and I am not anywhere near overweight as a result of eating properly the rest of the time.

The only potato I do not like is the couch potato. I think there is no excuse for someone who has all the time in the world to sit around and do nothing all day due to their lack of attention to their eating habits or failing to exercise for 20 minutes 3 days a week...

FOOD GROUP #12 - FRUITS AND JUICES

These are sweet and sugary sources of carbohydrates that are to be eaten only during AM hours and as a dessert of sorts, following most everything else. After a carbohydrate meal or all alone by themselves, they are most enjoyable, I personally think. If you are healthy and have your body fat under control, an all fruit, no added sugar jelly or jam is wonderful on toast, bagels, etc. Berries in my cereal are great too. But again, if you haven't been eating right, have dug yourself a nice, deep hole of belly aches through poor nutrition, then you may want to have fruit alone for a while.

Sweet grapes, apples, mangoes, kiwis, applesauce, figs (did you know every fig has a bug in it), plums, papayas, nectarines, plantain bananas, dates, raisins, cherries, pears, honeydew, cantaloupe and prunes, just to name a few (prunes increase intestinal contractions and bowel fluid secretion like phenolphthalein, the chemical used in many laxatives) are all fantastic in maintaining your digestive health. Potatoes and tomatoes are actually considered 'almost' fruits too you know! But these fruits aren't the same as acidic fruits.

The acidic fruits are oranges, grapefruits, pineapples, tomatoes, lemons, limes, peaches (actually peaches and tomatoes are low carbohydrate fruits), sour apples, sour pears, apricots, berries, and sour grapes... Sour things. Think tart. Like sweet fruits, sour ones should also be eaten after a meal, by themselves, and completely separate from sweet fruits and starches, if you have digestive issues. Eating acids with starches destroys the enzymes that digest those starches. That's why we also shouldn't have vinegar on grains, potatoes, beans... 4 ounces of fruit or a piece the size of a medium banana has 24 grams of carbohydrates and 100 calories or so.

Have fruit, but do not live off of it. You know, fruits are most commonly associated with cakes, pies, desserts, creams...

And there is a reason they are used in such sinful pleasures. They are high in sugar. Fruits contain essential nutrients no other foods supply but we do not need 10 bananas a day to receive them. You can have a couple pieces a day if you like, but making fruits the staple source of carbohydrates in your plan is only going to backfire on you. What about juicing?

Well, if you do drink juices, they should always absolutely be the last things you ingest after a carbohydrate meal ONLY (post workout maybe). Yes, I have heard it all before too. Drinking juices during a fast may relax your digestive system but they do not contain as much nourishment as the pulp left behind to produce them does. I do not care what nonsense you heard on TV from that crazy old guy with the bushy eyebrows. The magic of nature comes from eating whole foods, not raping them of their virtue. Natural sugars like pure maple syrup have a healing effect on the liver after it has emptied itself out all night long and depleted itself of glycogen. Blackstrap molasses works well at this too.

Having a tablespoon in my water upon waking is the closest you'll catch me at adding sugars to my diet. A glass of juice, around 8 ounces, has close to 120 calories and it's 30 grams of just plain old plant sugar. If you are drinking store bought juices, make sure it does not contain any added sugars similar to 'glucose solids' or 'corn syrup' at least. You'll overload your pancreas and make yourself FAT thinking it's healthy regardless of how healthy you think your selections are. Wine? One glass, every other day, mid-evening, after dinner is fine. But no more than that. If you want to argue the matter, you're a drunk. Just kidding. But do us both a favor; never drink to a point of intoxication. Soda? Please. Burping after a fine swig is enough proof the body is rejecting it so get a clue. And the glycemic index ratings, typically used by diabetics to gauge the rate their foods burn once eaten, are thrown in our faces more than they should be and are easily summed up too. This 'index' is only important to people who eat junk food.

The 12 Food Groups puts things into enough perspective for anyone to straighten their blood sugar levels out. Eat real food as often as you can and avoid processed foods. Period. So rather than worry about things like the glycemic index or eating one food over another because you are a diabetic, make sure you have several forms of carbs at a time or at least have them separate from your proteins and fats. For instance, if you have a banana, have a banana and a whole grain bagel. If you have pasta, have sauce and veggies. If you have rice, have soy sauce and beans too.

I question the glycemic index because it is based on studies of single meals, which provide insufficient evidence on which to base recommendations. The index takes no account of studies showing that the GI does apply in mixed meals. The index is a valid and potentially useful concept, but is also deceptively presented. There are a number of unanswered questions, and despite the objective that progress cannot be made without balance, balance comes from eliminating junk food.

I had a 235 pound 65 year old lady come to me once. She had been an insulin dependant diabetic for 50 years at that point. 2 months later, she was down to 205 and her doctor told us she no longer needed well over half of her insulin. She still fought me tooth and nail over the diet and ate twice what I asked her. This went on throughout our relationship. Yet, despite her convictions, the end result was still success. The 12 Food Groups WORK. She dropped 45 pounds of fat and gained 15 pounds of muscle during that time.

I can't tell you how many women I have encountered or that have emailed me who are guilty of eating just fruit all day in an effort to lose weight. Success is achieved by having combos of the 12 Food Groups, not by enjoying only one group a day. If you would like further information, please visit our website.

CALORIE COUNTING TIPS

1) Eggs: A larger whole egg (white and yolk together) contains about 6 grams of protein, 4 grams of fat and 60 calories. The white alone has 5 grams of protein and 20 calories and the yolk has 1 gram of protein and all the fat.

2) Seafood: Averages 23 grams of protein and 3 grams of fat per quarter pound (4 ounces).

3) Animal meats: Trimmed of visible fat and skin, contain on the average quarter (1/4) pound, almost 25 grams of protein, 5 grams of fat and 135 calories.

4) Organ meats: On the average, 1/3 pound or 5 1/3 ounces contain 20 grams of protein, 10 grams of fat and 170 calories.

5) Dairy products: Low fat cheeses have around 8 grams of protein, 1 or 2 carbohydrates, 5 grams of fat, and about 80-85 calories an ounce. Non-fat milk and yogurts are about 8 grams of protein and 12 to 16 carbohydrates per 8 ounces.

6) Nuts and seeds: An ounce (1 oz.) of seeds, nuts or nut butter contains around 7 grams of protein, 7 carbohydrates, 14 grams of fat and 182 calories. Some are higher or lower in these figures.

7) Fats and oils: A tablespoon of oil contains almost 14 grams of fat and 126 calories. Get your essential fatty acid oil from www.PerfectEFAoilBlend.com

8) Fibrous Garden Vegetables: Veggies yield around 2 or 3 grams of protein, 5 or 6 carbs and around 30 calories per 4 oz.

9) Beans (legumes): Approximately 75 calories, 4 grams of protein and 15 carbs per 4 ounces (oz). That's one fourth of a 16 oz can.

10) Grains: Grains and cereals generally contain 4 grams of protein, 20 carbohydrates, and 1 gram of fat per 110 calories.

11) Potatoes: Something the size of a medium potato (3 oz.) should have around 3 grams of protein, 22 carbs and 100 calories.

12) Fruits: 4 ounces or a piece the size of a good banana has 24 grams of carbohydrates and 100 calories more or less. Medium sized apples are usually 3 oz and contain 80 calories.

TAKING MEASUREMENTS THAT MATTER...

Ever had something important to do and you didn't write it down so you could remember? Ever let weeks, months or years pass by without getting something down? Start making commitments.

Tell yourself today, "If I don't put my goals down on paper, I am kidding myself. Goals are the reason we achieve success. They just need to be specific goals and the plan starts from where you are now, not from where you wish you could be. You will be surprised at how by simply writing your goals down and reading them, you will become motivated than ever before in getting them achieved. Success teachers have suggested it forever and for good reason. Let's see where you stand today.

Calves: Stand feet together, all weight shifted off the leg being measured. Relax. Wrap the tape around the thickest part.

Today: _____ Again In 13 Weeks: _____

Thighs: Measure both of them. Spread your feet about six inches apart and shift your weight to the leg not being measured. Be completely relaxed and tape the largest part. Don't be shy.

Today: ____ Again In 13 Weeks: ____

Buttocks: Stand up straight, feet flat, relaxed, heels together. Measure around the (gulp) biggest part off your caboose!

Today: _____ Again In 13 Weeks: _____

Hips: Same position. Keep standing. Measure just a little higher than the butt. I know, I don't like it either... Just do it...

Today: _____ Again In 13 Weeks: _____

Waist: Place the tape one inch above the belly button or around the largest part. Measure from the back and ['don't' ?]close your eyes!

Today: _____ Again In 13 Weeks: _____

Chest: Lift your arms out to the side at shoulder height and wrap the tape under your armpits. Let your arms come down again and relax.

The measurer should tape you right across the nipples all the way around. We aren't measuring lung capacity so don't take in a deep breath. Ladies, you know what to do here.

Today: _____ Again In 13 Weeks: _____

Shoulders: Tape around the widest part. Again, relax...

Today: _____ Again In 13 Weeks: _____

Upper Arms: Raise the arm to be measured straight out to the side palms up and keep it relaxed. Measure where it appears to be thickest and then do the same spot on the other arm too.

Today: _____ Again In 13 Weeks: _____

Forearms: Out of curiosity, go ahead and measure your forearms while you have your arm extended.

Today: _____ Again In 13 Weeks: _____

Body Weight: No one wants to admit they weigh more or than they consider optimal but get on that scale now!
It's IMPORTANT!

Today: _____ Again In 13 Weeks: _____

BODY FAT PERCENTAGES

Before you workout or do anything else today, including the reading of this chapter, your next step in getting up off your butt and doing something about looking and feeling better is to record those tape measurements. Yes the ones I just listed. See how big your various body parts are. Get your tape out, measure your parts then let's continue. This section of this book tells you how to use that simple tape measure for a VERY accurate means by which to determine your EXACT daily caloric intake needs. After thousands of clients, it's right on the target every single time. It's not how fat or built you are that determines your caloric intake. It is your lean body mass. So make sure that part is right first. Then forget what you think you know. This isn't as simple as your weight multiplied by 10 or 15 or 20 or whatever either. Despite the fact measuring your body fat this way or any other way is merely a guess, it is a good enough guess for now.

I already know that you may or may not think you are as fat as you should or should not be. I also know you may or may not know why you are as heavy or lite as you are today. It seems that many people believe the thyroid gland is a major key in fat loss. It may be, but it's what you do to the rest of your body that affects your thyroid and fat loss most. People also think dieting slows the metabolism and therefore the thyroid down. Others believe the marketing and seek the use of caffeine pills (diet pills of any sort) as their obvious solution.

Others believe surgeons who say if you are too fat or too thin, you should have your thyroid removed. The truth is, fat people have slow thyroids because they allowed themselves to get fat. Thin people do not have fast thyroids, they have poor eating habits as well. A fat person who becomes thin will find that their otherwise slow thyroid suddenly returned to normal after they lost the extra weight. Skinny people who begin eating better, put on a little muscle only to find that their thyroids have regulated too. You do the math.

Dietary habits interfere with the metabolism and slow the function of your thyroid. Weight problems are not caused by the thyroid gland initially not working right. Weight problems are caused over time by YOU to a point your organs fail. Face it. YOU 'made' YOU over or under weight. YOU also make yourself unhealthy. Overweight people tell me all the time that they eat less often than you think they do. They usually eat like a pig once a day, usually only at night, and starve themselves all day long. You know that's not good. Underweight people eat all the time but rarely do they eat enough, and that's their problem. Look, I had two sisters come in to my office both weighing 160 pounds.

They also each had 25% body fat which means they had about 120 pounds of muscle mass and 40 pounds of body fat apiece. They were twins and both told me they were to begin thyroid medication in 28 days as prescribed by their physician. Have you ever dieted but only got fatter? Listen to this then... One sister ignored my recommendations because she thought 'my' plan was nonsense. She didn't agree with giving up sweets, sodas, nor McDonald's French fries. She felt that protein powder was more important than fresh proteins, vegetables, grains, etc. She lost weight and went from 160 to 130 in 28 days.

The problem was, all her weight lost was in muscle. She now had 90 pounds of muscle (down 30) and 40 pounds of body fat (the same as where she started) at the 130 pounds she now weighed. This had her now at 31.77% body fat instead of the 25% she started off at! She looked AWFUL too. Truly obese and disgusting with all that loose skin and cellulite. Got cellulite? That is due to eating both table and fake sugars (chewing gum and drinking soda), not eating enough essential fats, nor drinking enough water. All the things she kept doing. Her sister on the other hand listened to what I had to say and although she only lost 20 pounds, it was all in fat.

It doesn't matter if she lost ALL the weight she wanted to, it matters that she did the right thing, she LOOKED REALLY GOOD and SHE GOT REALLY HEALTHY doing it. Going from 160 to 140 brought her body fat down from 25% to 14.3% (as opposed to the 31.77% her sister achieved by starving herself)! One of them was told by their physician not to start taking thyroid medicine. Guess which one... I will save the weight gain stories for another chapter. What you are about to read next will become the blueprint for everything you do regarding food intake for the rest of your life. Take it very seriously. Take your body fat percentage very seriously.

The International Sports Sciences Association says 5% of your total body weight being fat for men, and 8% for women is the minimum you need to sustain a healthy body. Are you anywhere near that low? They also say 10% for men and for women 15% is optimal (which I whole heartedly agree) and anything above 20% for men, or 25% for women is, I am sorry, just plain unacceptable. That's clinical obesity. Chronic obesity is anything above 25% for men and 30% for women.

Not much of a difference really. By the time you are above 20% fat, you're already worrying about what others think. I am sorry if you are in this group, I feel your pain, but please, do not turn back now. I am here for you. However, I want you to know the facts no matter how painful they are to hear. 15% for men and 20% for women may be comfortable for some, but as a whole, society has either made us far too comfortable with being fat. We are generally confused about how lean we really ought to become. Let's stick with 10% for men and 15% for the ladies.

This will get you to the beach without wearing dresses or t-shirts the entire time. How much body fat DO YOU have? Maybe you should get a professional body fat analysis performed and find out. In fact, have two or three done and "average" out the results. They shouldn't be more than $20 a pop. If they are, you can get skin-fold calipers instead, but that's not fast enough.

We need to get started today. So instead of thumbing through the phone book to see if someone in your area uses "Bio-Impediance" body fat (composition) equipment or professional skin-fold calipers (calipers measure pinches of body fat all over you to determine fat levels), let's act quick. What I need you to do right now is take 3 'before and after' pictures. Go ahead, grab a camera. Stand like a crucifix with your arms out to the sides and up at shoulder height.

Have someone take a picture from the front, from the side and one from the back. Make sure you are at least in the picture from your ankles to the top of your head. We need to see what you are made of, so wear revealing clothing, don't cover up. We will use these photos as 'before' and 'after' progress reports to 'witness' your progress. Take them by standing in front of a white wall wearing fat revealing clothing like short shorts and either no shirt or a sports bra (ladies are the only ones supposed to wear a bra or bikini top, yes, some jokers have sent me silly stuff in the past). BUT JUST DO IT. After all, you will never look like this again!

Embarrassed or not, you need proof! Later down the road, when you are being re-measured, photographed, weighed or whatever, continue to use the same scale, tape measure, camera, equipment or technician in order to maintain the integrity of your results. Deal? Ok... Do you know how much body fat you have right now but aren't being honest with us? Forget about scheduling a body fat test, we haven't that sort of time. If you do know your body fat %, great, if not, we'll simply use your waist measure.

With some of you, I realize that you may or may not have a lot of fat around your waist right now. You may be trying to gain weight instead of losing it too. I still want you to measure your waist for me. Is it what you want it to be? For every inch bigger than it is supposed to be, you have a good 5 to 7 pounds of fat to lose.

For instance, let's say there are 6 extra inches around your belly (or BUTT, if you store the fat in your hips and booty, measure that instead...).

Ladies, 6 inches of unwanted flubber is a good 30 pounds you need to lose in body fat for sure. It could be more, it could be less, but it's close. You know whether you are too fat or not without measuring but measuring the fattest part of your body, also gives us approximately about how much lean mass you have.

Knowing this information will give us a good indication of what your minimum daily caloric intake should be too.

Confused? Forget about it!

Fill out the following info.

1. Your Current Body Weight Is: _____ 174
2. Your Current Waist Measure Is: _____ 47 ½
3. Your Goal Waist Measure In 30 Days Is: _____ 40 __
4. The Difference Between The Two Measures Are: _____ 5.5
5. Multiply The Difference By 6: _____ 33
6. Deduct The Above Figure From Actual Weight: _____ 141
7. Divide Step 6's Result By Ten (10): _____ 14.1
8. Multiply Step 6's Result By Step 7's Result. _____ 1988
Step 8's Result Is Your Daily Calorie Recommendation.

330/meal

Next...

1. Divide Results Of Step 6 By Your Body Weight: _____
2. Subtract The Above Result From 1.000: _____ 19
3. Multiply The Above By 100. Your Body Fat % Is: _____ 19%

Again, like anything else, this is a guess but as good as any. No matter the results, do not eat less than 1200 calories a day.

WHY YOU SHOULD EAT SIX MEALS A DAY

Realize the caloric figure you come up with may seem higher than you have been eating OR it may be even lower. It is easy to recommend a fixed amount of calories (also known as energy) for anyone using this formula. This represents an estimate of what you need to survive efficiently each day on. Whatever you're doing now, adjust your calories to be closer to what we have come up with right here. It's important you do this.

Now that you know how many calories you are supposed to consume, divide those calories by 6. It is best for you to have the same amount of calories at each feeding right now, and six is the minimum number of meals you should be having each day. I know, "How could I possibly fit six meals into MY schedule?"

Easy... Breakfast, Brunch, Lunch, Mid-Day Break, Dinner and Mid-Evening.

If you want to or currently already eat more often than this, simply divide your daily calories by 7, 8, 9 or however many meals you plan to have each day. I often eat 10 times a day. Upon waking, on the way out the door, mid-morning, lunch, mid-day, mid-afternoon, dinner, mid-evening, before bed.... Wait. That's only 9! Well, whenever I have the time, it's alright to eat more often. Just don't OVER eat...

Eating more than 5 times a day gives you a metabolic edge over other people especially when those meals are all equal in calories. Rest assured eating 6, 7 or 8 times a day following this simple rule, you cannot become fat. There is no way on earth clean food in the right amounts can fatten anyone up especially if they follow the program every single day for even a month.

A meal every 2 hours is acceptable. Let's start right now by determining what your plans are for the next few hours. Are you at home? Are you out or heading out?

Will you have time to stop for food? Should you pack a snack to take with you? What did you eat last? Should the next meal be a carb or a protein meal? Do you need both because you will be out for the next couple of feedings or the entire day? Are you going to be working out? Or will you possibly be napping soon?

Are you trying to lose weight or gain weight? Too much to think about right now? No matter what runs through your mind when you think about eating 6 times a day, know that an hour should never pass without fresh food being already in or going in to the belly and this is the single most valuable habit you can adopt. You must give the body a continuous supply of nutrients for building muscle, burning fat, keeping your energy levels up and blood sugar regulated.

Face it. Your way didn't work or you wouldn't be here. I am an industry insider. I probably know something that you do not. You can't risk that I don't because odds are you only disagree because you haven't done this before. So how would you know? Trust me...

Ever had a hunger pang? Growling belly? That means the body has gone into a catabolic state because you're not eating often enough. Not good. That also means you are losing muscle, which in turn leads to the storing of more body fat. Don't like that fat on your back? Speed the metabolism... Eat something! You will notice that when you cut calories back on a typical diet you don't get hungry. This is only because you are mixing your foods the wrong way and they do not digest properly. Your meal just sits there in your gut, so you never get the signal that it's time to eat again. This is BAD.

One reason we have equal sized meals is to teach you that meals are not meant to be Holiday-sized feedings just to hold you over until you eat again but moderately sized and sensibly prepared feedings that your body can digest more easily. Keep your energy levels constant.

Several medium sized portions a day digest easily. Eating small meals one at a time adds up to more and more food by the day's end, which is better than eating everything all at once. There is no starving and no letting the metabolic fires from within slow down on you. This is key. Only eating one or two large meals to make up for your supposedly cramped schedule is unacceptable. Look where you are. You're not in your best shape. Admit it. We can all fit 6 feedings in if we WANT to... Let's move on. So, with that said, breakfast, lunch and dinner are not going to be enough to elicit the results even if you eat from all 'four' food groups and take your wonder supplements bought off the television. We need food and nourishment all day long, especially in the morning, so let's begin there.

Breakfast is usually skipped because people don't feel like eating or think they haven't time. Well, if you do not eat breakfast (especially before working out or within 10 minutes of waking, the body shuts things off inside of you to prevent excessive muscle or organ loss. This is the first thing you're doing wrong that leads to fat storage. When we starve, the body's priority is to protect your insides from eating away at themselves for the energy that they are not getting from food. Food, we can all agree, is what we were designed to run off, not out, of anyhow.

That's why we crave the stuff, get rumbles in the tummy and why I repeat it again and again so you will remember it. Without food, the body cannot do the things you want it to yet run efficiently... Let's assume then we were actually created to get our nourishment by leaching specific nutrients little by little from the foods we ingest. Foods are, for the most part, made up of carbohydrates, proteins and/or fats that happen to contain all the essential vitamins, minerals, amino and fatty acids you require for EVERY SINGLE HUMAN FUNCTION there is. This is stuff we all understand. It is also common sense that if you want fully nourished, you MUST try to eat all sorts of different foods at some point during each day.

'o not always provide what we need however. This is why
add certain supplements to the diet. We can also
that in order to get enough of the essential nutrients, we
ould be required to ingest more food than we have time for too.
Sure, I bet some of you already do eat six times a day but having
bird-sized meals followed up by feasts doesn't count for much in
this scenario.

If you aren't 100% completely certain you have control over how
much, what time, and what specific foods you eat at one meal
opposed to another, you had better become so today. We need
carbs, fats and proteins just to make it through a day. The
sources of those nutrients may vary. On occasion, what we think
is nourishing us is really leaching from us or feeding the toxins
that make us tired, sick and fat.

I cannot twist your arm to eat more food and to do so more often.
You are correct about that. However, oddly enough, without
enough calories there aren't enough 'macro' nutrients (carbs,
fats, proteins) so all your expensive supplements, which
hopefully contain all 'micro' or 'trace' nutrients, are most often
useless. When I first began eating right, I hadn't any idea eating
the correct amount of food each day would make a difference
either. I would wake up, eat a box of cereal, chug a gallon of
milk, boil a pound of pasta, eat 3 pounds of fish, and by the end
of the first few days always ended up quitting because I only got
fat in the process. After that, I would panic and eat only a can of
tuna the first 3 meals of the day then wonder why I was losing
muscle. So yes, I know what a yo-yo diet can do to your
appearance first hand.

Do you experience any of the following after eating: Mental
grogginess? Yawning? Falling asleep in class or at work?
Thoughts begin to cloud? Choose your words wrong? Nasal
congestion? Hives? Belching? Well, times are about to change.

Now you're listening? Well, I've got another analogy for you...

Let's pretend you are a car. You pick the car. But like an automobile, does it make sense to try and drive without gasoline, oil or transmission fluid in your engine? No? We agree there. Good. Then why would you insist on low quality products to run it or blindly mix gasoline and oil together into your engine at the same time? The body cannot produce the enzymes to separate fuels by itself.

You need many different sorts of fuel to operate a car, but a car doesn't store each component in the same areas, nor can it separate them to save its parts if you mix the wrong fuels together. And if you want your body's fuels (food) to digest efficiently, you DO NOT mix them incorrectly either.

No matter how low fat, low carbohydrate, high protein, vegetarian or wholesome your eating habits are.... There are rules to be abided if you want control of your health and appearance. Besides having at least 6 meals of equal caloric intake, you must always be certain to keep carbohydrate foods away from your protein and fat foods. Carbohydrates require neither fat NOR does protein require sugar to assist in it's digestion. In fact, these nutrients inhibit one another's usage. If you eat protein with starchy carbohydrates, one goes incompletely digested.

Thus, the feeling like a basketball is sitting in your gut after you eat them together (like a cheese burger). The myth that you need carbs and protein together for additional glucose in your blood to transport the digested amino acids is unfounded. Most of the sugar used to transport protein comes from previously eaten carbohydrates, not from what's eaten at that particular meal! Carbs spare your amino acids and proteins from being used as energy, only if you eat them separately. Otherwise, protein doesn't get used efficiently at all. Sure, most all carbs have some protein in them. However, the protein that nature provides in a fruit, vegetable or grain does not have the same biological composition of meat or fish protein.

It's obvious there is a chemical difference between an egg and oatmeal or they would be the same thing. One is from a plant, the other is from an animal. With that said, keep your proteins and fats together and clear of added starchy carbohydrates. Fat plays a major role in hormone production but only ends up wasted when eaten with carbs. Contained in all protein foods, like meat and eggs, there is always a little natural fat in whatever we choose to eat.

As mentioned in the 12 Food Groups chapter, you should trim the skin off the meats you eat, toss aside the marbled fat, then add healthy fat back to your meal... Protein naturally requires fat to assist in its digestion, and that's why all protein sources in natural forms do contain fat, but the skin unfortunately isn't the best source of quality nutrients. Not interested in hearing that? Who do you know on a low fat diet that is not doing so well? If you eat no fat, the result is always poor hormone levels. That means little to no muscle growth for men, difficult menstrual cycles and blotchy skin for women and very little fat loss for every body. Signs of protein deficiency.

And so you know, protein with a little fat eaten a couple hours before bed will increase your natural secretion of growth hormone in response to a decreased blood sugar level that occurs naturally as you enter into sleep. So eating late at night is 'good' for you after all... That is if you ate SIX meals the same day beforehand... Many of my top models and bodybuilders do this... I know what you're thinking, but there really isn't a comparison to eating right and having a plate of spaghetti and meatballs before sleep...

Did you know that you could take a pill with different enzymes to break down different foods, depending on what you wanted to eat? Well, the body does this for you. The enzymes that act upon carbohydrates are not the ones that act upon proteins and fats and vice versa. The pharmacies who make your over the counter enzymes know this, your doctor knows this too.

CARB MEALS VS. PROTEIN AND FAT MEALS

For some reason, no one told you to eat accordingly. Instead, they simply made a pill available. Taking digestive enzymes with your meals is like admitting you are doing something wrong, but you aren't sure what. It's nothing more than a band-aid, which you can swallow. Is that natural? No. Am I sure of this?

Yes, I am 100% absolutely sure that carbohydrates require different enzymes than protein. Look up alpha amylase, sucrase, etc. which all break down carbs and then look into the various peptidases for protein like trypsin and chymotripsin, you'll see what the truth is for yourself. One thing is for sure, you'll discover that metabolisms are completely separate and different for these different foods. It is very possible you went to school or have researched this before but haven't seen anything to indicate that only one set of enzymes or another can be released at a time in your belly. You either overlooked it or depended upon whatever your trainer or favorite magazine said instead of looking it up on your own. Research it again.

It'll be right there in front of you. Trial and error, along with actual footwork, takes a person a long way. My path led me to the conclusion we were made this way intentionally. I haven't a clue why we were created to digest food like this but it seems most religions agree, food was made for man, not man for the food.

So, I am pretty certain our bodies were designed to digest what was prepared for us ahead of time. And even if not, we can at least agree that plants and animals, while both contain life, are completely different things. Almost any medical doctor will admit, carbohydrates require a completely different metabolism and set of enzymes to digest than proteins do. Ask one. They should be able to at least confirm that the release of hydrochloric acid (in the stomach) lowers pH to a level (below 3.5), which inactivates alpha-amylase (one of the enzymes which break down carbohydrates) to allow protein to better digest.

This alone lends credibility to my program. If they can't, they either haven't paid attention to their nutrition and digestion or as I said, they possibly overlooked it. An obvious sign your foods aren't digesting properly is GAS. Agree? Well, just bear with me, follow the program and if after 30 days on the Know How the gas is GONE, then it's safe to assume with those results you are making some sort of progress. Right?

Upon chewing the first bite of food at breakfast, the necessary enzymes to break down your food of choice are secreted and become present in the gut all based upon what the food is recognized as by the brain. Once this meal is eaten, it pushes whatever is left in the belly from the previously eaten 'last' meal, meat for instance, through the duodenum into the small intestine. Other enzymes are then secreted (like tyrosine and chymo-trypsin) in order to deal with scavenging your previously digested mush for amino acids and fats. This is why you shouldn't skip breakfast even if you're not hungry. The lack of hunger comes from food still being in the gut. It needs moved out so the body can do it's job correctly. No, this isn't when you poop it out, but it determines whether your metabolism is up to par.

Metabolism is the process where cells either create through anabolism or destroy through catabolism. Catabolism is the process of living tissue being broken down and turned into energy or waste. This is destructive. Anabolism is the process of construction. You want the body as anabolic as possible to burn fat, build and maintain muscle and speed the metabolism... So keep eating... Because of breakfast, that protein meal that you ate last night is now pushed into the small intestine and is being absorbed into the blood stream. Amino acids from that food are being distributed throughout the body to build and repair tissue (this is what is meant by maintaining a positive nitrogen balance when dealing in protein metabolism). But that's not all. This process of getting breakfast in, so the remnants of last night's meal goes down, also pushes yet another meal from the day before, into the large intestine.

The process of pushing the food all the way through requires yet another meal because you can store two or three meals in your backside at any given time. Most studies done on digestion were performed using people eating a variety of foods together, not separate. This is why they say the basic reality boils down to carbs digesting faster than proteins, which digest faster than fats. That's true, but that's from mixing foods and giving the body no other choice and why it takes a 'normal' meal 6 hours to leave the stomach unless you put something on top of it to push it through.

If for no other reason and to avoid constipation, PLEASE do not skip meals no matter what happens. If you feel you won't be able to eat on time, eat sooner, never later. Skipping meals leaves food inside of you to rot. That's not good. If you do not listen to your body, food can sit in your digestive tract long enough that it actually begins to spoil.

This is part of the reason you stink so much when you break wind or eventually do go to the bathroom. Stinky, putrid food has been clogging up your digestive tract. You receive little or none of the nutrients you are expecting to from letting this happen. They will die in there before ever getting to be absorbed if you do not eat in a timely fashion. Remember, the stomach is merely the first stop. That same food must somehow next exit the gut and enter the intestines to begin nourishing you. Not only is it a waste if the food cannot continue this simple trek, but the spoiling process is what creates the toxins that make you sick, tired, stinky and slows your metabolism down.

Sad thing is, it really is such a simple and easy process to assist along. You just have to eat another meal. If not, it will be the accumulated toxins from years of bad eating habits that slowly and quietly poison you to death. Ever heard this story before? "But Joe was just over to the house last week. He didn't have cancer." YES, he did. It wasn't found in time because not only wasn't he getting checkups but these things catch up to you.

Once they do, you're in trouble seemingly over night. It's too late now for Joe. You however can make change NOW.

He's dead at age 38 from colon cancer. Are you ready to extend your life or did you want to go pick out your coffins and headstone instead? It's that serious. All that fat, saggy, blotchy skin, and lack of muscle means inside, you are dying. Literally dying. I don't care if you are 16 or 60. You're killing yourself. Wish you could be like you were when you were younger and hate what you see in the mirror, especially when you are naked? Well, do SOMETHING like EAT ON TIME. Assuming it takes 1/2 hour to finish a typical meal, and you could easily schedule your meals 3 hours apart, waiting 2 and a half hours after finishing a meal is about average time to begin eating again.

If you aren't hungry this often, now you know it's because THERE'S UNDIGESTED FOOD IN YOUR GUT waiting to be pushed through. The stomach rarely empties on it's own efficiently. You just think it does because eventually you get hungry. So, humor me, just in case something doesn't get efficiently digested from the previous meals you ate, it is always a good idea to make sure it gets pushed through your digestive tract anyhow. Think of the food in your stomach as a clog in a sink or toilet drain. Substantial forces must be applied to move what's clogging the pipes down and out your drainage (and in this case, your digestive) system.

You'll always be 'clogged' or 'backed up' unless eat on time and ingest equally sized meals. This leads me to my next point. If you do not have bowel movements regularly, you are in more trouble than you realize. FULL bowel movements are normal if performed more than twice daily. Dropping pebble sized 'poops' do NOT count as 'going' to the bathroom. No matter what you believe causes your constipation nor whether you think it will go away on it's own, eat something. Eat something again in 2 and a half more hours. Eventually, you'll go to the bathroom regularly again.

PIECING IT ALL TOGETHER

RECAP: One meal goes in the belly. A second meal pushes it through to the small intestine. A third pushes it into the large intestine. A fourth pushes it almost out of you. If you are eating enough at those first 4 meals, it may have pushed through. If not, 5 meals should. 6 meals always does....

And for heaven's sake! ALWAYS chew your food slowly and thoroughly (with your mouth shut and lips together please)! Your stomach has no teeth. If you're still getting gas, that is why. Sure, there is the possibility you may be drinking too much water with your meals too, but either way, chew slowly, keep your lips closed, digest well, excrete it out, repeat...

Six meals merely optimizes things so like most healthy people, you can experience a couple healthy movements a day. No, I do not mean you'll have diarrhea nor to offend you with all my poo poo talk. Understand, if food were meant to stay inside of you, there wouldn't be a means for it to come out. Nor would we be so uncomfortable when it doesn't. I used to think 3 meals were all you need. That's how I was raised. But as I got older, I craved mid evening snacks more and more often. When I began working instead of sitting around all day, if I didn't snack between meals, I couldn't function. As each meal or snack was added, the better I looked, the better I felt. Eventually a seventh meal was added and I will never eat less than that again. You can start with six...

What you should do now is determine the amount of food you are eating currently and see how it compares to those new caloric allowances we figured a few pages back using your waist measure. Take a moment and feel free to write in the book, it's yours. Try to figure up how many calories you are eating on an average day by jotting down, meal to meal what you ate today on a separate piece of paper.

Do this tomorrow if you must. Do it for the next 7 straight days too. Separate your foods, begin to eat more sensibly and take notes of everything you do from now on. Because guess what? We need to know what you're doing, how your appetite fluctuates and what your preferences are. Why? As you build muscle and eliminate fat, you will be required to eat more and more calories in order to maintain what you build and keep the results coming in. If you do not know what you are doing, how will you know what needs to be changed? Maybe you think you know... At least this way you'll be certain.

It's all about meal preparation and we are about to discuss the RIGHT way to set up a dietary road map. To start, we already know your measurements, we know your body fat percentage, we know your calorie intake and we know how many calories you need per meal. Next, we'll schedule four of your meals (or snacks) to come from the protein and fat foods we discussed in the 12 Food Groups. Metabolism is the process of every cell to either create anabolism or catabolism. It is also the process by which food is turned into useable substance by a human being. Catabolism is the process of living tissue being broken down and turned into energy and waste. This is destructive.

Do your best to eat proteins and fats at a 3 to 1 gram ratio to one another and include green vegetables. Some people think this diet has them eating less protein because we only have it 4 times a day instead of at all meals. That's not true. Because you get to eat more when you do have it, you're consuming plenty and because digestion is enhanced, more protein is actually absorbed. Not satisfied? Add a fifth meal then. But continue to have it separate from your carbs.

Others ask if 4 meals are too much. No, it is not. Take your lean mass and divide it by 3. However many pounds that is, say 180 divided by 3 is 60, then that's how many grams, 60, you should have at your 4 protein meals. Add it up at the end of a day and there is PLENTY but not too much.

Divide that number of grams of protein by 3 and that is how many grams of fat should be eaten with those meals too. It's perfect. I wouldn't ask my grandfather to begin eating 240 grams a day or even the 60 grams per meal eating that much requires. But I would if he were a bodybuilder, maybe, depends on his weight. However, no matter who you are, if you eat your protein and carbs together, you might really be assimilating half of what you think you are.

With protein containing 4 calories a gram and fat having 9 calories a gram, that's 420 calories if I eat 60 grams of protein and 20 grams of fat at my protein and fat meals. I tend to have 500 calories per meal these days so adding 80 calories of say, spinach, will round my meal off perfectly. To get 60 grams of protein from nonfat cottage cheese, I will need to have a little over 2 cups which is 320 calories. This leaves me with just enough room to add 20 grams of fat from Lemmon's Oil before running out of calories. I would then just make up for not having greens by having them at another meal. Sounds like a lot of fat though doesn't it?

It really isn't when it's a healthy fat like flax seed, butter, olive or Lemmon's Oil. If I haven't convinced you to increase the fat a little, at least keep the carbs separate and maybe go with a 4 to 1 ratio instead. Do not exceed your allowed calories no matter what you decide. If you are a vegetarian, search for high quality, low carbohydrate, protein alternatives at your health food store. It's alright that you choose not to eat red meat, fish or chicken. That's fine.

I do feel eating some farm fresh eggs and organic cheese with your tofu is only going to help you in the long run. No matter the choices, round the meal off with a nice bowl of green vegetables. Next on the list, plan another two feedings as carbohydrate meals. If you do not feel like eating a lot of carbohydrates, cut back on them a little, but no matter what, always keep them separate from your protein and fat meals.

Understand, you are supposed to HAVE CARBS. Limit yourself by only having two meals if you like, but do not neglect them entirely. Whatever you heard before about low carb dieting in the past, FORGET IT. It's all nonsense (for the most part) and I want you to go select items from Food Groups 8 through 12.

The hardest part of this program is reading all of the food labels of every food that you purchase before you eat it and trying to learn what the foods really are made of. Considering that any 6th grader can read a cereal box, this really shouldn't be a problem. Serving sizes DO vary quite a bit from manufacturer to manufacturer and should never be taken for granted no matter how many foods you memorize. The calorie counting at first will teach you to eat for satisfaction, not out of pleasure (gluttony). The reading of labels out of curiosity at least will make everything else seem like a piece of cake.

How many carbs are actually contained in your carb meal depends upon what foods you select. Some foods are higher or lower in protein content than others and this is what affects the amount of carbs they contain. For example, fruit doesn't really have any protein per 100 calories but a potato has around 3 grams. Beans contain 6 or 7 grams, rice 4 or 5, and some grains have up to 10 grams per 100 calories. So you see, this varies the carbohydrate contents anywhere from 15 to 25 grams depending upon what you're eating.

This is why you should always read labels. Especially if you've taken up carbohydrate counting as a second hobby... I don't want to give the impression that you have to count calories for the rest of your lives however, walking around with 4 extra inches around your gut doesn't look good. And it's not right. But by counting calories as in counting what you take in, not in limiting yourself, you will learn where to begin cutting the calories (or raising them) if necessary. You need this info to be certain you are feeding your lean muscle tissue enough to burn fat.

Forget about limiting carbs or falling into this percentage or that percentage. It's really not about the carbs being in a "ZONE" or below 30 grams a day that counts after all. It's about scheduling 6 meals a day and making sure 4 are protein and fat (low carb) based and that 2 are carbohydrate (low protein, low fat) based. For you Zone followers, I want you to know right now that for every pound of lean body mass you change or are different from the person next to you, there is a coinciding change in not only the amount of calories you ingest, but the basic structure of those calories and the mixtures in which you receive them! The percentages of protein, fat and carbohydrates are rarely 40-30-30 folks. Begin tallying up what you already eat and count those calories as accurately as possible if you haven't already. See if you're really in a zone at all.

This is how easy eating 6 times a day is... We all go to sleep at night at some point. We all also wake up eventually, so that's breakfast time. We all work, even if it's around the house each day, so, mid-morning, take a snack break. We are all either allowed, given or know we can take a 15 minute break. That's enough time for brunch. We all also get lunch breaks or can at least make time for one, even if it's 30 minutes later than planned. We all can. So do that too. There's 3 meals already...

Mid-day is when we all take our second shift breaks or can at least sit around long enough for a few moments to snack again. When I was a district manager of a health store chain in Los Angeles, I used to have my snacks in my car while driving. So I know you can pull it off. And I haven't met a business person yet who didn't gain the respect of his peers by making sure they took care of themselves by having a snack on time. Not one. Eventually, we all come home from work or we prepare a dinner of some sort wherever we are. We also get a craving mid-evening or sometime before bed, so eat something then too. Still not convinced? Come on, take charge for a change!

When I was in the Army, I would wake up first thing in the morning and have a glass of protein powder before heading out to do PT. After our hour-long session of pushups and running, I would go stand in line at the mess hall for an omelet and cottage cheese. On the way out, I would put bagels and bananas in my larger pants pockets to snack on and hold me over until lunch. At lunch, I ate a lot of burger meat, pork chops, cheeses and veggies. Before I left the mess hall again, I always grabbed apples and muffins for the mid-day snack. For dinner, I had more meat and veggies before cleaning up to hit the gym.

After my workout I would go to the grocery store or commissary to get a quart of nonfat milk to drink. Now of course, you can argue it isn't so easy doing this sort of thing while out in the field or playing war games in the woods. But if you're smart, and I know you are, you'll know better than that now. It's as easy as you want it to be. Another time I worked 2 jobs while studying for school. One was from 12:00 noon until 4:00 p.m. each day and the other was a 11:00 p.m. to 7:00 a.m. midnight shift. I ate at 10:30 before work, 1:00 a.m. on break, 3:30 a.m. at 'lunch' and 6:00 a.m. before the boss came in.

I would get off at 7:00, be home at 7:30 a.m. and sleep until 11:30 a.m. As soon as I would wake up, I ate and left for my second job. I ate again at 2:00 p.m. then was off work at 4:00 p.m. and back in bed from 4:30 p.m. to 6:30 p.m. I ate when I arose at 6:30 and then from 7:30 to 10:30 p.m. I was either buried in studies or going to the gym for an hour each night. Which ever it was, I ate again at 8:30 p.m. between courses or after the workout. At 10:30 the cycle started over again. Man, I needed a nap though. I was always tired.

While in the Army, I dealt with lack of sleep. If it were wartime, or if an emergency arose, you would need deal with that lack of sleep so we literally slept deprived ourselves as a form of training. But you will still 'feel' it eventually if you do not get your '8' hours of sleep each night. Sure, you can ignore the signals.

But once you realize that the first 2 hours of sleep you get must be fully uninterrupted if you want your hormones to regulate and that actual healing doesn't begin until after the body has been down for 6 hours straight (and that only lasts for 2 more hours), then you might try a little harder at getting to bed EARLIER instead of LATER each night. One night with poor rest affects even the best of us for days at a time and the accumulative damage can be devastating.

In fact, in my one apartment I had this horrid cricket that seemed to like toying with me by doing all this blasted chirping only during the times I was trying to sleep! Not while anyone else slept, JUST WHILE I TRIED TO! So to ensure my 8 hours of rest, I wore earplugs. How funny is that? No, coffee and artificial stimulants will not make up for a lack of sleep. Do not use caffeine pills when you are sleep deprived unless you want ulcers later in life. And early morning isn't a good time for stimulants anyhow. As far as proper timing goes, your adrenal glands are weak in the morning but strong midday. But that isn't mid-day every-day.

You can drink coffee only 3 or 4 times a week maximum without stressing your adrenal system. No? Do you get tired after a cup of java these days? Gee, your adrenals are falling apart and it's time to cut back. Thank God this only lasted 8 months of my life. I was sleep deprived, felt like a vampire but was doing better than anyone else I knew on such a schedule. Since I only had a 4 hour shift to work from 3:00 a.m. to 7:00 a.m. on weekends, I made up my lost 10 hours of sleep over weekends.

I always ate my 6 to 8 meals a day plus I worked out 2 or 3 times a week and got my rest. So no excuses. You have time. You just have to make it. The point is, it doesn't matter if you wake up at 4 o'clock in the afternoon because you work a midnight shift. Whatever time you arise, immediately begin eating 'breakfast' or whatever you want to call that first meal. Breakfast is the start of your day, the 'breaking of your fast' so to speak...

So eat something! And continue to eat again at least every third hour you are awake, even if you are awake 36 hours in a row. Eat on time, no excuses. You can vary your feeding times, if necessary, catering to your work, sleep and exercise schedules, but anyone can at least make sure they are fitting in 6 meals and 6 hours of sleep each day (although 8 is best).

You know I am right. But it still sounds like too much trouble to you, eh? Look, if your primary excuse for failing to stick to this program is your laziness to pack a lunch or prepare and control your own food, or counting a few calories, and you insist that Met-rx or EAS powders are better for you than real food, then failure is your own fault. Don't EVER neglect to use the 12 Food Groups as a guide and NEVER under eat nor have less than 6 meals a day. TRUST ME ON THIS ONE. You can sit around all day and blow off exercise.

But don't you dare tempt fate by shoveling tons of food down your neck NOR starving yourself believing that you won't get fat from it. Excess is excess and starving yourself shuts the metabolism down. And every day you put off exercise is another day that you will look in the mirror and complain about your fat gut, the cellulite, the bags under your eyes, your tummy pouch and everything else you secretly aren't too proud of. No, I am not psychic and I do not know you individually, so I am not personally assessing your condition. I do know how most people are though. I can't say how long it will take to correct what's wrong in anyone, but a day worked is a day gained, isn't it?

Do not write me and tell me this program failed you, I have made it as simple as anyone ever has right now. Only YOU can FAIL YOU on this or any other program. I, nor 'it', can fail you... The KNOW HOW is designed around how "Nature" works, not some marketing campaign and therefore I assure you, it cannot fail unless you refuse to accurately follow it! No amount of kicking, scratching, arguing or bogus propaganda is going to get your digestive system to work any better than I have explained it.

I will say it until I die, if you aren't separating your foods, NO program will work for you! Well guess what? There is logic in everything you have tried before...

Low carb diets <u>are</u> only partially successful because they separate the carbs from the protein and fat sources (even though the diet eventually fails you because you DO need some carbs...Only not with your proteins and fats). If you are following the Atkins diet and have no muscle or have sagging skin, thank the good doctor who prescribed it... There's no saggy skin on this program.

Low fat diets work a little but it is only because they separate the fats from the carbs The failure of these plans stem from having your essential fats eliminated, eating too many carbohydrates and the fact you were still mixing proteins and carbs together. Have acne or menstrual issues? Still fat after months of effort? Have unbearable gas? Three strikes, you're out! If you mix your foods, you're going to end up protein malnourished. This only occurs when one, it isn't digesting or two, you're not eating as much protein as you should to begin with.

Most of the emails I get are from people telling me they already 'know how' to eat a 'healthy' diet and they 'look great' too, but in reality they are exaggerating or they wouldn't have contacted me to begin with. I look at their diets and it is amazing how many carbs people eat with their proteins. All the Zone Diet does in an attempt to remedy the high carb or fat deficient approach is cut your carbs in half by merely making it look as though you're doing something beneficial. Nothing more, nothing less, and it's obviously not enough. Like the vegetarians who have been mixing fats and carbs together forever, you become overweight or sickly looking despite lowering your calories. It's not from a lack of protein, it's from mixing fats and carbs. I have had a lot of people tell me that they are on 40-30-30 Nutrition based program like the Zone that suggests eating chicken, rice and broccoli with a little olive oil too.

I have just as many tell me that in the morning they have something like oatmeal with egg whites and maybe one yolk... You know the routine. Steak is a no-no for a low fat dieter though. Well, once either of them made the simple transition to having oatmeal and rice at separate feedings from the eggs and chicken, that's all it took for the magic to begin. I don't mean simply separately eating one bowl and heading to the other.

I mean eating 2 or 3 hours apart. Is it too much to ask for you to eat potatoes separate from steak if that means you're allowed steak again? But does the diet really work for everyone? Is it all things for all people? Yes it is. In fact, it even works for animals. Listen, do you have a pet? Well, I do. When we got him, he was 2 pounds. 2 years old and full grown. He's a half Chihuahua and half Jack Russell mix (don't ask, I don't know) but he was a little guy. 6 months later, he weighed nearly 6 pounds.

No, he didn't look malnourished when we got him, and no he doesn't look fat today. Since eating better, giving him vitamins, minerals, oils and good food, he is a completely different dog though. All we did was put him on our diet. Tequila (his name) eats proteins at one meal and grains at another. So does our other little one, Teaka, a teacup Chihuahua. She's 3 and a half pounds. The veterinarian told me that her breed doesn't normally exceed 2 pounds. What can I say? She eats right. Meats, vegetables, fruits, real food. So does my 3rd dog, Pookie. It amazes me how people can malnourish their dogs by feeding them 'dog' food and then wonder why the little guys are so full of ailments. But what's worse is that you do it to yourselves.

Unwittingly, we are malnourished, yet overfed and so unhealthy, but you don't even realize it. Another automobile analogy (can you tell I grew up next to a General Motors Plant?)... What is wrong with those people that go out of your way to put premium gas in their cars and regularly change its oil using, once again, only the best supplies? All that fuss...

But when it comes time to fueling up and cleaning out or adding the best ingredients nature has to offer to their own bodies, it's a different story. They still eat fast-processed, ready made, fat free foods and write off being fat, sick and unattractive on genetics. Proof is in the pudding. Speaking of pudding, I suppose if we expect them to actually get with the program we better give everyone some more ideas of what to eat! Write down what you ate today because you're going to need this info in a minute:

Breakfast:

Brunch:

Lunch:

Mid-day:

Dinner:

Mid-Evening:

Other:

Supplements:

Notes:

WHAT TO EAT AND WHEN

For breakfast, if you want carbohydrates (meaning you have decided upon having a low fat meal consisting of no meats or fats, only starches and fiber filled carbs), maybe you'll choose to have cereal, nonfat, NOT whole, 2% or 1%, but nonfat milk, and follow it up with a piece of fruit. You could even have a slice of toast with no sugar added jelly or nonstick pan fried hash browns with fat free butter on the side if you like (just do not fry the potatoes in oil or use real butter because carbohydrates can't be eaten with added fats). You could even have pancakes or waffles instead if you prefer, using pure maple syrup in small amounts, fresh berries and nonfat butter. Again, we don't use real butter with carb meals.

If you don't feel like carbohydrates, have a protein and fat meal like eggs and bacon with a side of diced mushrooms, onions, and peppers. The vegetables are essential and assist in digestion, eating just protein and fat alone will eventually backfire. In fact, you can treat yourself to a REAL OMELET using these guidelines. Take onions, peppers, mushrooms, broccoli and a piece of real cheese and place them in the fold of some eggs and you're all set! This then, is a perfect, animal source, protein and fat, therefore low carbohydrate meal. Remember, fibrous carbs are not the same as starchy carbs.

What about lunch? Have pasta if you want it! It's not evil. But because pasta is made of grains, it is a carbohydrate food, so instead of having it at dinner when carbohydrates are harder to digest for most people, have it earlier in the day, here at lunch when the body can more easily handle carbs. Make sure to not use any oil, butter or meat on it. You can still have all the garlic, spices and diced veggies you always do, but use nonfat sauce and nonfat Parmesan cheese instead. On the side you could have garlic bread made with non-fat butter and fresh garlic, however, meatballs are to be eaten at another meal all together.

If you do decide to have meatballs, make sure they aren't made with bread crumbs (that's a starchy carb, a no-no with protein foods). In regards to nonfat butter, I do not mean margarine, I mean fat free butter. I assure you, non-fat butter exists. I get mine as a spray but there are other brands that come as spreads. Ask your grocer which they carry.

An alternative for lunch could be a bowl of rice, with black or red beans and steamed veggies on the side, topped by soy sauce. Do not add oil or meat to this dish either. It's a carbohydrate meal, so keep it low fat. You can however use nonfat broths to flavor the rice. Remember, 'non-animal based' meals of carbohydrates are to remain as low fat and vegetarian as possible in order to allow for proper digestion. You can only have carbohydrates with other carbohydrates.

If you do not feel like carbohydrates for lunch, have some roasted chicken with a salad. You can use REAL cheese plus a little REAL dressing because low fat and nonfat dressings all contain sugars (which are carbs, and a no-no with meats). Also, you cannot have FRENCH FRIES with this meal either! Potatoes are carbohydrates and frying them in fat is a bad idea. Chicken and salad... That's a proper 'animal based' protein and fat meal!

TIP: I normally have salads when I go out to eat. Most people order their lunches from restaurants. This is important to note because a restaurant sometimes delivers extra food that exceeds your allowed calories and other times they add things that are off limit to your meal. Just because they do this doesn't mean you have to actually eat the extras. Keep your protein and fat meal low in carbohydrate. No fries, no croutons, no rice, no baked potatoes with meat...

You can have a potato with your rice or pasta meal anytime you like, you can even have it by itself, but you cannot use butter or cream (unless it is non-fat) and carbs are off limits to all protein meals.

I order my potatoes 'dry' and take them home with me for a snack or something later. DINNER. You're always better off having fish, poultry or meat with steamed vegetables or another salad at this meal. Again, have your typical steak and potatoes dinner but without the potatoes! That means you're allowed more steak, so who loses with that sort of deal?

This plan goes for your kids too. Do not use the excuse that your kids want to eat different. KIDS EAT HOW YOU TELL THEM TO. Get used to eating this way then figure out on your own (you know them better than I do) how to get them on the program or they will be unhealthy and worried about their appearance when they grow up too. If you allow that to happen, you're an awful human being. I truly feel that way. My child's health means the world to me. Not having control over what your kids eat, like in the case of separate households, is one thing. But if you have any say so whatsoever, enforce it. You know what is right or wrong. Forget about the high self-esteem that comes from looking trim and fit… Without good health we have nothing.

What we have done to this point is cover your three main meals. Breakfast, lunch and dinner. Next, let's discuss your snacks. Plan on eating one between breakfast and lunch then another between lunch and dinner and one more between dinner and bedtime. Keep one rule in mind when selecting a snack..

You can't have two carbohydrate feedings in a row.

Having two carb meals in a row triggers a negative chain reaction inside of you that tells the body to burn muscle tissue and store fat, which is obviously undesirable. Interestingly enough, having two protein and fat meals in a row, is optimal, because it gets your body burning fat and building muscle. For this reason, I schedule one carbohydrate meal in the AM (either breakfast or brunch) and the other lunch or mid-day, depending on when the first one was eaten.

So, for snacks, if your breakfast was full of carbohydrates, you should have protein snacks of cottage cheese, or almond butter (no sugar added) mixed with whey protein and Lemmon's Oil on celery at brunch. If breakfast was protein and fat based, then a snack of bagels and fruit would work. But if you have carbs mid morning, you can't have them at lunch. In my opinion, breakfast and lunch are the best times to have carbs.

Mid-day, if lunch was a carbohydrate meal, you could have coffee with heavy cream, pure whey protein and spinach or broccoli to follow down the hatch too. It's a good habit to always have greens in the freezer at home or work if need be. Sure, it sounds crazy to eat greens at every meal, but it works wonders on healing your gut and clearing the intestines. If I had protein at lunch, like a salad I ordered from a restaurant, this is when I will eat my baked potato that came with it. I sometimes get an extra potato or bring a bowl of beans for these 'meals between meals'.

Mid-evening. I cannot insist upon you're eating a mid-evening snack often enough. Mine is usually scrambled eggs, but I always have a protein meal as a final feeding. It speeds the metabolism like you'll never know unless you try it for a few weeks.

TIP: Never have more than one whey drink a day and never use a meal replacement powder or protein bar. The body was designed to run off food, not cookie dough and cake batter... If you only use what I recommend then you cannot fail. If you eat any other supplements, I cannot assure you of anything.

All those high protein, low carb bars are junk food too. If it tastes like candy, it is candy. If it isn't, then prove it to me. Don't send me sales literature as though that's some sort of proof, it isn't. Send me actual proof. You can't. And like it or not, there isn't a single bar that's as good for you as real food and since most 'health food' bars are made by candy companies anyhow, you really haven't a clue as to what's in them (glycerine IS a carb).

At best, your 'meal replacements' are nothing more than expensive after-workout snacks. It is 100% absolutely true that you can become firm WITHOUT magic potions, protein powders and caffeine tablets.... Forget what the ads say! Throw it all away! Get a refund! Why would the 'establishment' and supplement salesmen want to hide things from you? Because if you knew the truth it would put an end to a billion dollar business.

You wouldn't visit a fat farm clinic or QUACK doctors that peddle things like Phen Phen if you knew the truth so these companies suppress the info that would otherwise deter you from their services. It would also put many pharmaceutical companies out of the picture. In their defense, most companies haven't even a clue what they are doing to begin with. It's just big business to them. That doesn't make it better, but it does explain a lot. Dishonest people are driven by the all mighty dollar and many of the folks out marketing the hottest fat loss products available only know about, you guessed it, making money. Not nutrition. Not exercise. They have made their livings their entire lives telling people what they want to hear to sell anything from floor cleaners, car wax and protein powders.

REMINDER: Breakfast is best eaten immediately upon waking. Lunch can be eaten at what you determine is your regular time. Dinner too can be eaten at your regular time. However, this is important, Brunch has to be eaten half way between Breakfast and Lunch. If you eat at 7:00 a.m. and 12:30 p.m. then Brunch should be scheduled in the middle at 9:45 a.m. Your Mid Day Snack is then also eaten half way between two meals, Lunch and Dinner. If you eat at 12:30 p.m. and 6:00 p.m. then schedule this snack at 3:15 p.m. right in the middle. Your Mid Evening Snack is then to be sandwiched half way between Dinner and bedtime on non-workout days. Say you're normally having dinner at 6:00 p.m. and hitting the hay at 11:00 p.m. then you must eat a snack at 8:30 p.m. nightly.

DIET SURVIVAL ADVICE

My pre-workout meal is usually nothing more than my protein powder, coffee and cream. It may be steak and spinach. If I am in a rush, like first thing in the morning, it's definitely protein powder and cream because I need it fast and I would never workout on an empty belly. I will also save the carbs for after the session. Keep your caloric requirements in mind.

The 12 Food Groups give you plenty of different items to select from but the foods listed aren't the only ones you are allowed to eat. No way. There are a wide variety of other foods to choose from that fall into those same categories. You can use almost any one of them to devise your own diet and wean out of old eating habits, just compare notes. If you make sure you've paid attention to what the appropriate food categories are at all times by using the 12 Food Groups as a lifestyle guide, you cannot fail. A goose and a squirrel may not be the same things as a steak or a chicken, but they are certainly the same type of foods. They are protein and fat sources.

Nuts and seeds aren't the same, but they are close. If you don't like nuts, have seeds instead. Just review the food groups when necessary and you'll be fine. In fact, email and ask me anytime if you get confused. By following these diets over the next 13 weeks you will not only get yourself into shape but you will possibly discover tastes for different foods you didn't know you had. However, you may not be so open to new things and want to change a particular item here and there. That's fine. All menus are interchangeable. If you do not like a particular food, then go to the 12 Food Groups and select another one from that particular 'group' to replace it with. If there is a carb you don't like, replace it with another carb. Exchange protein for protein, fat for fat, etc. etc. Even if you want to have a different protein meal one week that you saw on another one of the menus, simply switch it with the protein meal on your current one, or carb for carb, etc. and so on.

Sometimes, certain foods may even seem a bit expensive, depending on the season, and other times, you'll change a meal because you're eating on the run. I understand.

Just stick with the 'like' for 'like' idea. Replace carbs for carbs, proteins and fats for protein and fats. As far as expense goes, I used to get canned tuna instead of fresh tuna and sometimes we got green beans instead of broccoli. For the most part though, you will discover that foods bought at a store are much more affordable than the ones at restaurants. Fish is fish, red meat is red meat, beans are beans, fruits are fruits, but not if you buy them at a gas station or restaurant instead of a grocery store. Stick with the most natural sources of food you can afford, whenever you shop and all will be fine.

How practical is this plan? When we go grocery shopping, we grab a couple containers of oatmeal, a gallon of nonfat milk and a few bags of frozen berries for breakfast. That is about $12 for a week's worth. We also get seven 32 ounce containers of nonfat cottage cheese to mix with one and one half tablespoons of Lemmon's Oil. At $2.50 a container and a third bottle of oil (10 servings) for $4, that's another $20. A bag of rice and a bag of beans, plus a little bouillon and soy sauce is $5 at the most total for the week. We have cream in our herbal tea during the afternoon with a can of tuna and that's about $5 a week for the fish and $3 for cream.

Next we get some chicken, steak or salmon, a pound a day at no more than $2.99 a pound, a little container of feta cheese, lettuce and mix it at home with one and a half tablespoons of Lemmon's Oil for dinner. That's $30 a week maximum. Eggs and broccoli are the last meal so we grab seven bags of 99 cent veggies and seven 18-packs of eggs for $1.50 each. That's $18 for the week. I suppose since we use 2 bottles of multi-nutrients a month too we can call that another $10 a week between us. Add it up. That's basically $60 a week for an athletic man for both food and supplements. $200 a month for food, $50 for supplements.

See, it's extremely practical. So, start today with whichever menu you want, even if you configure one of your own based upon likes, dislikes, budget or convenience. Do not forget, each meal is to be equal in calories. Only you know how many calories a day are required if you've done the math earlier in the book. Divide those calories by six and that's your per-meal allowance. You did do that didn't you? I wrote this book for you because I wanted you to use it to succeed. But all I can do is explain things to you using the best methods I know.

I still cannot twist your arm to do the foot work. Besides, if I get hit by a bus, this book and the prescribed homework is all you'll have to remember me by. So depend upon yourself. Not me or anyone else. I cannot guarantee your success unless you can guarantee that you will take appropriate action. I do not know what you are going to do with what I gave you, but one thing is for sure, do not expect anyone else to make the changes we've discussed for you. This is YOUR gig and YOUR gig alone.

Anytime you need a reminder or an added bit of motivation, feel free to write me, but read and reread this book as often as necessary to commit it to habit. You know what's in it for you if you do. You'll become healthier and successful. I didn't settle for less than that myself when I started so now it's your turn to get on the ball. You have already set a goal for yourself and now it's high time you began working to attain it. How long will it take to reach your goals once you start? That depends on your current condition. You could gain 20 pounds of muscle in 40 days if you need it or you could lose 100 pounds of fat in 6 months if that's what is necessary. All things take time, but fortunately for you, not as much time as it would using other methods. Just remember, no added sugars (like in juices and canned products) or processed oils (like in peanut butters and processed cheeses) or fake sugars (in gum and fat free products) or any of these un-natural additives in anything you buy from now on. No, this doesn't limit your ability to eat flavored foods.

You will discover that even by adding just a couple of spices to a meal, you can experiment with virtually anything to flavor your meals. I sparingly use sea salt (which contains dozens of minerals and will not cause water retention) and ground black pepper on almost everything I eat. I love garlic too and I eat a lot of that, but it's a preference to smell so Greek! I also like 'hot' stuff like spicy mustard (wasabi) and chili sauce. We love our spicy cheese dips, soy sauce, low sodium broths, unsweetened catsup, yellow mustard, and steak spices are all great to keep on hand. If you aren't familiar with some of the spices I have listed, that's alright. Your grocer should be. Ask a clerk at your store where to find them.

As far as cooking utensils to prepare your foods, most adults should know how to cook (although I am never surprised these days at how many people do not know the simplest of things). I get by using plastic measuring cups, spoons, knives, forks, plastic containers, bowls, plates, a microwave, blender, frying pan, spatula, boiling pot, strainer and a big stirring spoon. Some of you might want more than this. If so, pick up any other items you may find listed in a recipe book or that you learn of somewhere else the next time you're out shopping! I have a peanut butter maker and rice cooker myself. That's about as exotic as I get. If you are still one of those people who say there is no time to cook, mass prepare your food twice a week. There, no more excuses.

Some things like oatmeal or scrambled eggs I cook the same day, but I might crack my eggs the night before or dice my veggies twice a week. I will grill chicken and steak once a week but make my broccoli daily. I refrigerate or freeze whatever I cook that that won't be used for a few days then simply pull it out and microwave it when I want to eat. Another example, we make soup out of virtually anything we can buy from the produce section of the grocery store. We use beets w/tops, carrots w/tops, garlic, celery, parsley, garlic, okra, squash, garlic, water, more garlic, onions, meat... boil, add garlic and then we eat!

It's a soup that not only tastes good, but cleans our systems out as well. It's easy to make and if frozen, lasts as long as we need it. So get off your but and cook some food! Preparing your own meals can be both easy and fun plus awfully tasty if you pay close attention to the ingredients you choose. Using sensible flavorings on even foods that you normally wouldn't go near could end up making them some of your new favorite dishes.

Beware, it is possible to add too much of a seemingly innocent ingredient and destroy the taste of an entire meal. if you dump too much salt on a pasta dish or if you add oregano to your oatmeal or by adding sugar to protein. This is most likely because far too many companies out there slip bleached sugars into our foods and spices. You better begin reading EVERY THING before placing it on your food or in your mouth. You CAN learn from your mistakes. Become aware of your every move. So if you add sugar to a protein by accident, that doesn't make it acceptable to eat. You can't digest a protein with sugar on it efficiently.

For example, one morning, I added cinnamon to my whole fat cottage cheese and the particular brand of cinnamon I used had sugar in it. I ended up throwing it all out. I also refuse to put sugar on anything including my cereal and coffee. Sugar literally disrupts your digestive system. Just about every spice you find at the store can be used with the exception of products with added sugar. Look at what you have now in the cupboard to see if all your choices truly are sugar free (artificial sweeteners are off limits as well).

If you feel the need to use any sugar at all for a recipe, you should only use the purest sources possible, like real honey, maple syrup or unbleached raw cane sugars... Even that white fructose which is sold in 'health' food stores is bad. So do your best to cut back in all areas of added sweeteners.

Sugars tend to cause ALL other foods containing them to ferment in your gut and remain undigested. That leads to all sorts of other degenerative disorders. Reversible disorders, yes, but that's no reason to subject yourself to the torture to begin with. Your best bet is to avoid all sweet and "white" colored food products to begin with so there is nothing left to question. If you want to use sugar just because you think the taste of real food is boring, GROW UP.

Get used to eating without additives for a change. Use little spicy twists and you can make any 'bland' old food taste more "socially appealing." If you're only excuse for cheating is because of taste, spices are one of the safest and most cost effective preventive measures against cheating. Refusing to eat 'right' because things aren't 'sweet' enough is sure evidence of your chemical addictions to food. Try cooking at home on your own today and you'll see! Just watch what you put in your mouth. Common sense dictates that if bacteria won't digest a cup cake then what makes you think your stomach will? Who can deny the exciting fringe benefits here?

You get to continue to eat whatever it is that you already do eat, but somehow, this program magically allows you to succeed for a change by merely separating your foods into appropriate meal patterns. How could ANYONE have a problem with that? You're going to eat what you want to anyhow! At least with me, you're allowed! You would have to be insane to not give it a try! The same foods you like to eat now, only at different meals.

Some flavorings will change calorie intakes. With that said, don't forget to count your calories, watch your grams of fat, carbohydrates, and proteins closely, and read the labels of everything you put in your mouth from now on. Most food labels list serving size (measure), servings per container (how many), calories per serving (you may be having more or less than one serving so read this), total fat (per serving), total carbohydrates (per serving), and total protein (per serving).

Also read the actual ingredient list. Hydrogenated anything or syrups or sugars or stuff ending in 'ose' is a no-no. Only YOU can watch out for YOU.

I want you to succeed. But I can only show you how. I cannot force you to do what I recommend. I hope you do not expect anyone else to make the changes for you. YOU make change and the people around you will make change. I know some of you have been blaming everything and everyone around you rather than looking to yourself for the source of the problem. Try taking some initiative. Stick out your chest. Hold up your head up and be willing to get your hands dirty. If that is too much for you right now, give this book to someone who is ready to put their past behind them and restructure their future. I WAS LIKE THIS TOO at one time! You're not alone!

What then should you expect to experience once you begin? Well, at first, you might experience some discomfort. I know, that's not a good feeling. You'll think the devil got a hold of you and that Don Lemmon is the patron demon, but stick it out anyhow. Your metabolism is slow right now. It takes a few days, maybe even a week or two for your body to regulate its sluggish behavior. This has nothing to do with salt. Sodium isn't related to holding water unless you haven't been using it for a prolonged period.

Sooner than later the bloating will disappear on it's own but only if you stick it out. Just divide your age by 3 and that is about how many days it should take for your body to adjust to eating properly. By then you will not only 'know' the program is working, you'll 'feel' it and SEE IT. Either way, keep in mind the bloating is all fairly typical. You WILL drop body fat during this 'grace' period, despite the fact you're 'feeling' otherwise. What causes it? The bloating is caused for the most part by your backed up bowels. No worries, just relax, within a week, that will change. You will start noticing positive changes in your regularity and feel fine once the metabolism speeds back up.

Whatever you do, DO NOT QUIT due to this bloating! If you quit, every single time you try to start the program over again, you will bloat ALL OVER AGAIN! The bloating is a false feeling that the program isn't working. Just ride it out for the time being and no matter how nasty, oily, gross and fat you feel, ignore it. This is the body's only means by which it knows to dump toxins and shift into metabolic over-drive. It's like taking your car up a steep hill. It's tough going up, but once you're at the top, it's always a breeze coming down! Besides, you can literally vary your grocery list any way you like from now on. You picked the foods. You can even increase the variety in your diet using the rules we have learned so far. If all you're doing is eating what you always have, but you haven't seen any change until now... Things inside of you are FINALLY changing... So don't blow it by quitting. I don't care if you're bloated all month. Stick it out. I simply ask you watch what you eat and that you refuse to have junk food any longer. Not a single physician on Earth is going to say that's asking too much. In fact, talk to one. Your physician will agree with everything written so far...

Eating clean, exercising regularly, drinking fresh water, sleeping longer, only taking supplements that include vitamins, minerals and essential fatty acids and sticking with it the rest of your life... What's not to agree with? If your doctor says my diet sounds like bull, ask him to see his abdominal muscles. Are they visible? What kind of shape is your 'doctor' in? Can he out run most people his age? Out weight lift them? I think you can tell if their advice is worth taking or not regarding this matter. If they tell you that it's normal to crave hydrogenated oils and artificial sweeteners, that chlorine in your water is fine, a lack of sleep and exercise is acceptable, or that junk food is 'OK' by them too, it is time to switch doctors! I cannot begin to tell you how many elderly people have seen their cholesterol come under control or how many teenagers saw their pimples disappear by simply dropping the junk food and following the instructions in the next chapter to get those poisons out of you even faster. I have plead my case. Now get started.

DETOXIFICATION

In case you do not think that constipation or bloating has anything to do with making progress... Or your grandparent's cholesterol problems... I hope those of you who think constipation has nothing to do with many of your body's ailments and are living miserable, limited and inactive lives are only going to get worse in elderly life, if you make it that long. You will more likely die an early death. If you didn't look as bad as you do now 20 years ago, what will you look like in another 20 years?

Young and old, male and female alike, hear me now... If you do not have large, full and 'healthy' bowel movements regularly (twice a day...), then ask yourself, "Am I sure I am eating ENOUGH food?" Because no matter what you believe causes constipation or, like far too many people believe, that it will go away on it's own eventually, step one is eating more food.

If you want to feel better than you do now and know you need cleaned out on a more regular basis, all you have to do is make certain you are eating enough food for the most part. I assume you're already going to separate your foods correctly, but skipping meals, not eating your vegetables and cutting the calories back doesn't help you in the bathroom. That is unless of course you want stinky, milky, pasty, blotchy, dry, purple-ish looking, and easily bruising skin. Do you have high blood pressure, oily flesh, mid-day headaches or plan your day around potential bowel movements that never happen? These are all sure signs that you're still 'backed' up even if you do 'go' every day.

Ever wonder why some people you know look like they have aged 20 years in under a decade? Sure, they may be smokers or drinkers or what not, but grandpa didn't go from hearty and healthy in stature to bony with a bloated abdomen for any other reason. He is literally full of crap from his years of constipation.

Even if you are young, even if you have nice abs, if you have a bloated gut like a gorilla, you too are full of intestine clogging feces.

Your health is going to get really bad because your immune system can't fight the toxins in your bowel fast enough to defend the rest of the body in this condition. You lose muscle and your belly only gets bigger and bigger as the colon loses more and more control. I spent a lot of time on the crapper straining my brains out from as early as I could remember to as late in life as being on this diet full time. I would get gas so bad as a kid my parents would sit me on the toilet and wouldn't let me leave until there was evidence in the bowl that my bowel was empty. I was there so long at times my legs would fall asleep. I continued struggling with my movements until I was 21 or 22.

I know, that's not something any of us want to admit, but if I can do it, I think you can come forth too. It's time we do something to remedy the issue. Let me tell you something else, it's not what comes out, but what is left behind that hurts you. What goes in must come out. Think about 'that' for a moment. If the body was supposed to store it's 'waste' inside of you, there wouldn't be a process to drop it out your backside to begin with, and it wouldn't be so uncomfortable for you when it doesn't. No, it's not 'normal' to struggle to have a bowel movement.

If constipation, diarrhea or the feeling you're giving birth every time you want to go poo-poo has been plaguing you, it may be time to give mother nature a hand. No? Well, what you're doing now isn't working is it? Listen to your body. It's giving you a subliminal message. "Clean me... Clean me..." Seriously. The colon needs to be cleaned inside and out. Just to make sure we erase the errors of your past, I suggest you begin by performing a regular series of daily enemas for a short period of time. Don't kid yourself.

If you are constipated, you are toxic, and the fastest route to detoxifying the body after straightening the diet up is by giving yourself a good pipe cleaning. Sorry, fiber supplements aren't enough to solve your problem. Fiber helps to prevent further constipation, but if all you needed is 'more' fiber right now, we wouldn't be here. Why doesn't it? Because fiber doesn't dislodge what's trapped in there. It merely gets the fresh stuff past the crusty parts. The solution? Go out to the local drug store today and buy a half-gallon enema bag. It looks like a hot water bottle. Ask your pharmacist where in the store you can find one and do not be embarrassed by it.

Later the same day, when you're all alone and have your nerve worked up, fill the bag with 7 cups warm water, 1 cup freshly brewed coffee and hang it from a towel or coat rack near the toilet. Yes, that is 56 ounces of water and 8 ounces of coffee. Keep saying to yourself, "It's a bath for inside my butt." The caffeine goes in and 'challenges' -as they say- the liver to release it's backed up funk and bile. Bile is useful in many ways, but it's not meant to be backed up. Bile is supposed to emulsify the fats in our foods and is also a means by which toxins are eliminated from the body. Sometimes it just can't do it and usually it is because you're backed up. Are you burping, belching or bloated after you eat fats?

This is not only a sign that bile is backed up but now its led to having gall bladder problems. Not good. This can become quite serious, especially if you live in a polluted community. If you work or live in a polluted environment (which can be anywhere these days), things are absorbed into the lungs when you breath and then get dumped into the liver. This organ is sort of like the oil filter in your car and it wasn't meant to be abused. Things get worse when your community uses a lot of chlorine and fluoride in its water supply. After you eat, drink and breath the body is supposed to efficiently pull toxins out of your blood and mix them with bile to be carried out through the 'regular' digestive process.

Sometimes bile gets backed up because the metabolism has become sluggish. This is why your skin looks so awful, your breath is so bad, and most everything else including your joints may be ailing you. You're toxic and enemas are the easiest way to get your system going again. You see, bile is composed of salts, cholesterol and lecithin (the latter two are essential fats). When hydrogenated oils, which are bad sources of dietary cholesterol are eaten, they throw a monkey wrench into your bile's mix.

Usually good cholesterol is turned into a bile 'salt' which thins the mix. Hydrogenated oils are found in non-dairy creamers, lards, margarine and creamy peanut butters. When these fake fats are produced, it is done so by destroying natural foods, chemically converting them to longer lasting substances the body was never designed to digest. In fact, most countries in Europe BAN these things because they are so harmful to us. Some bile salts are secreted into the small intestine and eventually reabsorbed after circulation by the liver again. This could be good or bad because the enzyme 7-cholesterol dehydrogenase is regulated by the amount of salts returning through this process.

The more 'bad' salts that are made from 'bad' fats and the more that are secreted, the more that are reabsorbed, the slower the production of 'clean' salts from 'good' cholesterol becomes, and the higher your bad cholesterol levels increase. All because you're backed up and there is no 'exit' route for the waste to excrete itself properly. The conversion, circulation, production and excretion process of bile, toxins, cholesterol and waste depends upon eating, sleeping, fluids, anti-oxidants, b-complex vitamins, essential fatty acids... AND.... Taurine (taurocholic acid), glycine (glycocholic acid), copper (which are all found in large enough quantities in the Don Lemmon Multi-Nutrient for this reason). The final point there is that the efficiency of the body's ability to keep itself clean is not only based upon your regularity, but what you do to enforce it and what nutrients you are missing.

This is why sometimes you get diarrhea and sometimes the bowels look green. The green is the bile finally dumping itself out and the diarrhea is the body liquefying your bowels to squeeze what waste it can out through your clogged pipes. It's disgusting to think about and it's irritating to remember the last time it's happened, I know. But this is only happening because we aren't taught anything about proper bowel movements growing up, in school or by our physicians. It is a forgotten part of the health care system and it's why our children are having their appendix removed so early in life (or at all). The body knows it must keep itself clean even if you try to keep it backed up all the time. But it's not 'normal.' For now, if it happens, let the diarrhea pass and allow the body to eliminate itself the best it knows how. Take NOTHING to stop it. You have to let yourself clear out 'naturally' this one last time.

Now is not a time for fiber. Again, fiber allows you to go easier NEXT TIME, but it doesn't get what's trapped inside of you out. If you want a good fiber choice for later, select a barley fiber, as this is a great source. Psyllium will do too however, just don't think by using a fiber supplement, all your problems are solved. They aren't. What about taking medication? No, drugs are not the answer. Drugs only make you even more toxic. If the body breaths in toxins, if you are eating toxins, if you aren't 'regular' and you aren't getting any healthier, don't you get it?

It is your bowel movements that are limiting the removal of excess waste, cholesterol and toxins. So, let's clean you out. In order to perform an enema properly, the hot water bottle part of your bag must be hung high enough from a rack or wall that the water can flow downward through the hose at a relatively good speed. Pressure is important. It is second in importance to making sure the bag is secure from wherever it hangs so it doesn't fall! And always hang the bag near the toilet. You don't want to fill up with fluids then need to walk very far to let it loose. Once that is in place, you will lay on the floor, on a towel, on your back with your knees bent up and your feet close by your butt.

Practice doing a few hip raises from this position. You want to make sure you're situated properly. You want in a stable position where you can raise your hips and shake them up and down a bit with your feet still flat on the floor once the water is inside of you. The combination of warm water, coffee and shaking it all about is what dislodges old decayed feces from inside your intestines and prepares it for excrement. Think of it as shaking a jug full of water to clean it out. It's the same thing.

Once you're full, you will also want to massage your stomach around the abdominal wall muscles, probing deep inside the tissues to 'coax' the fluid through the intestines. This also helps the coffee go higher up inside of you to stimulate the bile release we just discussed. Now, how to fill yourself up... Of course, you will want to lubricate the hose nozzle with oil or a water based lubricant to allow for an easy rectal introduction. Do the same with your anus. Lubricate it. And don't feel funny about it. You are simply taking care of your much neglected health.

In case you fear an entire half gallon bag of water will cause you to explode, there is not only a clip near the end of the nozzle that controls the release of the water to begin with, but most people can hold a full gallon of water without trouble. Just make sure you let a little water run through the hose into the toilet so the air is out of the way before you put the tube inside of you. Once it is in, let the water flow inside of you gently, always controlling the flow using the clip on the hose. Of course there will be some discomfort, bloating, cramps and contractions. It happens until you're cleaned out efficiently.

If the cramps become fierce, simply pause the release of water and relax a moment. Take a deep breath but do not move too quickly during the contraction or you will shoot water all over the place. Poop will certainly follow it! So once the cramps disappear, don't stop the enema, but begin adding more fluid slowly. Eventually, you will be using the whole bag each session.

At first, maybe you'll only use a little before you give up, but you still need to come back and do this again anyhow. Not taking a whole bag is just a sign you're full to the rim in there. If someone tells you this process only cleans out the lower intestine, let him or her know two things.

One, a half gallon is too much water to only fill the lower end of your colon. And two, at least your lower end is clean while theirs is still... Well, full of it... You get the picture. You can put it off, but once you begin to realize you're not getting out of this what you put into it, so to speak, I want you to begin doing these enemas daily for 30 straight days. Then, do one every other day for 30 more. After that, do an enema every 3rd day for a month and in the fourth month, just twice a week is good. I would make sure I perform a cleansing once a week after that, usually before bed.

Detoxification IS something of the utmost importance if you want control of your health, let alone your appearance. All of us are toxic and each of us in different amounts. However, the differences between us are: 1) Our individual ability to naturally detoxify ourselves based upon our eating habits. 2) Our total exposure to contaminants and our intake or lack thereof in essential dietary nutrients and 3) Regular hygiene practices that assist in the otherwise sluggish natural cleansing process. Other common symptoms of being toxic include feeling constantly tired, aggravated, or just plain miserable (possibly because you are FAT and BLOATED too, but being overweight is a sure sign of being backed up o matter what you're willing to admit).

Eating right. Is it all about fitness, vanity or health? I spent most of my younger years wanting to attain some very cosmetic goals for myself too. But along the way I saw everyone I knew tearing themselves apart on their quests for a better body. Fitness is the ability to meet the regular demands of your lifestyle more easily and doing so with enough energy left over for the unexpected moments when we really need it. I like being fit.

I like eating right and health is something that goes without saying. But maybe we are really just in this for vanity? Usually that's it and well, I like seeing my knees while looking down towards the floor too. You can only do that if your belly isn't blocking the view. I have said it a million times and I will say it another million times before I die, make health your #1 concern and vanity, your reason for probably being here, will come full circle.

Of the many health challenges that we face daily, problems with the digestive system are the most dangerous and that is why this book focuses on it. Imagine what would be the result if a city's sewer system became so backed up that it actually failed to work at all.

What would happen if sewage pipes got so plugged up that they EXPLODED internally? We wouldn't see what's happening from the outside looking in under most circumstances but it would at least begin to leak gasses and stink. It's not just a bucket of acid in your gut. Some people think if you stick your hand down there, it will be melted within seconds.

Watch the Discovery Channel once in a while. Scientists have been sending little cameras into the human gut and rectum to view the different foods we eat as they get digested. Lord, it's not a good thing to see what is left behind. Take a sandwich for instance. Meats were sometimes visibly left behind when eaten with bread and potatoes. Meat eaten alone however was more often than not, disintegrated to a point it wasn't even there. Hey, the lady who performs our high colonics claims she has never seen foods go through a person as well digested as mine is.

My clients report their technicians state they've never seen people hold as much fluid either. That means we are not only processing our foods but we aren't holding any in our intestines. It's a testimony you may find bizarre but hey, I am not the one with digestive disorders...

When you eat your meat with your rice, tell me what you get. GAS. Sometimes AWFUL and foul smelling gas. Gas is indigestion. Undigested foods are what cause gas. In-digestion does not mean you only have a stomach ache per se. IN-digestion means something did NOT completely digest and it is complicating your digestive tract. Ok, so some of you think eating like you do doesn't cause health complications because you do not get headaches, intestinal cramps, bloated, gassed, or whatever, you're OK.

Sorry, you're still deteriorating inside, like it or not, and it's not normal to look the way you do. Sometimes the body shuts off your natural distress warnings like pain signals in your gut because you continue to ignore them. But the cause of those symptoms silently remains. I do my best not to laugh when fat, disgusting, chain smoking, alcoholics or otherwise disturbing people who ignore health criticize me for getting sick if I do. I just nod and ignore them. I can't get mad, and I do feel bad, but sometimes you just got to shake it off. You can't reason with some people. They do not realize if you get sick, that means the body is discarding an illness. It's fighting it off and winning. If you don't get sick, guess what, you are HARBORING the illness. The body is incapable of getting rid of it so it's just sitting in there eating away at your organs. Nice. P.S. When you do get sick, try some PURE honey. It eats away at so many strains of bad bacteria, including the ones not side tracked by antibiotics. Plus it doesn't hurt your good bacteria one bit.

My first enema came as a child when I went to the hospital for constipation. My second came when I returned the next year complaining of belly aches, which the doctor said was just constipation. The next year, I was back in the hospital again for another week's worth of probing. You think that's gross? What do you think the nurses have on their minds when they need to do this for people who won't take care of themselves. A year later my appendix almost burst.

WORKING TOWARDS SUCCESS

I am still thinking about that last chapter. A new doctor said if I would have had fiber and laid off the cup cakes I might not have had those problems. Hey, I was only 9 and suffered for 4 years waiting for that advice... But he remained our family doctor...

I know you want to be a healthy, vibrant, efficient and productive person. If you are not that type of person currently, odds are you are supporting that lifestyle. Admit it. If I seem intolerant, I am. And I do not feel sorry for you. There is no more time for that and there is no more time for worry, television, or any other waste of energy either. I do not tolerate whiners, excuses, or quitting. Success is from within.

Take one day each week to figure up what your actual diet was for that past week. Use your average total daily calories from the past seven days to determine what you must schedule for the next seven days. For instance, you may have scheduled 1800 calories a day last week but when you review the entire week when it's all said and done, you might have ended up with more or less here and there day to day. Your average daily intake might actually have been 1700.

Maybe you got fatter this week. I told you not to eat too little or that's what would happen. Maybe you ate 2000 instead of 1800 on the average because you cheated 3 times and that is what made you fat. If you under ate or over ate and got fat, go back and start again at 1800 calories a day for next week. Maybe you ate 2000 calories and made great progress. Stay at 2000 for this week then too. After this, add your calories as suggested each forthcoming week. As we progress, you will notice that you've become more and more tone by building some much needed muscle as you burn off all the unwanted fat (that's how the body is supposed to work).

Once the muscle is built and fat is dropped however, neglecting to feed your new lean body weight is what allows it to disappear and revert back to being fat again. Building muscle speeds the metabolism, losing it slows it down. This is why if you do not eat on time, or eat ENOUGH at ALL times, you become FAT! The body goes into 'ketosis', which is the breakdown of amino acids (muscle protein) for continuous energy. This is what you do to prevent any future headaches... Each week for the first 13 weeks on this program, I want you to ensure progress by adding a few more calories to your diet every seven days. You read that correctly.

Women 5 foot tall generally are able to get down to 100 pounds and remain extremely healthy. However, a good weight for a woman 6 foot tall is 150 pounds. So technically, to determine a good weight for yourself, a woman would add about 4 pounds for every inch over 5 foot tall they are.

So, 5'0" = 100 pounds. But 5'1" = 104, 5'2" = 108, 5'3" = 112, 5'4" = 116, 5'5" = 120, 5'6" = 124, 5'7" = 128, 5'8" = 132, 5'9" = 136, 5'10" = 140, 5'11" = 144, and 6'0" = 148 or so and etc.

Using this scale it will also be obvious what your hips or dress sizes should or should not be at these particular body weights. Ladies, ONLY YOU know your optimal size... And understand, hips aren't what they were at age 17 if you are now 25, 35, 45 or 55. This isn't because of fat, but increased bone density. That's right, brittle bones come from bad habits, not just because you age. Bones are actually supposed to get thicker and stronger as you age but you aren't allowing them to because you've been eating all wrong. Keep this in mind.

Men do well assuming 135 pounds at 5 foot tall and 225 at 6 foot 6 inches is normal. Actually, this may be a little thin for some of you but remember, Bruce Lee was only 135 pounds at 5'7" and Michael Jordan is 216 at 6'6" so you're not far off using this scale.

This means to assume a good weight for yourself, add 5 pounds for every inch over 5 foot tall you are to 135 pounds.

So, if you are 5'1" your optimal weight = 140...

5'2" = 145, 5'3" = 150, 5'4" = 155, 5'5" = 160, 5'6" = 165, 5'7" = 170, 5'8" = 175, 5'9" = 180, 5'10" = 185, 5'11" = 190, 6'0" = 195, 6'1" = 200, 6'2" = 205, 6'3" = 210, 6'4" = 215, 6'5" = 220, 6'6" = 225 and so and etc.

A safe waist measure would vary from 29 at 5'0" to 38 inches at 6'6" as well. That's 1 inch larger in waist measurement you are allowed for every 2" taller than 5 foot you are. I am 5'10" which is 10" taller divided by 2 = 5 and so my waist should be 29 inches plus 5 inches = 34" (and it is).

So, if you are 5'1" your waist measure shouldn't be bigger than 29 and a half inches....

5'2" = 30", 5'3" = 30 and a half, 5'4" = 31", 5'5" = 31 and a half, 5'6" = 32", 5'7" = 32 and a half, 5'8" = 33", 5'9" = 33 and a half, 5'10" = 34", 5'11" = 34 and a half, 6'0" = 35", 6'1" = 35 and a half, 6'2" = 36", 6'3" = 36 and a half, 6'4" = 37", 6'5" = 37 and a half, and 6'6" = 38 inches.

Yes, I am certain these figures are accurate. If you weigh the suggested weight and have these waist measures, odds are you are anywhere from 8 to 12% body fat. Some of you are built a little different but guys, like I said to the women, you know if you have an inch to lose or not and you also know if you are over or underweight too. I haven't met you, so you make the call. Point remains, as we progress, you must begin adding calories to maintain your results. If you are pregnant, wow, you're in luck! You get to add even more food than this! However, keep in mind, while it takes more calories than you're eating when not pregnant in order to create a healthy baby, you do not require all the extra food in one sitting!

Pigging out leads to fat babies and no they aren't supposed to be fat! Your child will grow up craving what it was fed in the womb so BE CAREFUL. Do what we just discussed and add only a few extra calories a week gently, as not to overload you or the child. On a weekly basis, over time, simply by adding calories a little as we go, you will feel like a Queen all the way up to welcoming that new addition to your family.

You may start off at 1600 calories a day but by the time Junior comes around, you'll have easily doubled that and kept your body fat levels under control all the while. I understand that as your hormones fluctuate, you may have cravings for the oddest of things. This is only due to a malnourishment of minerals, essential fats or proteins. Other diets, like those that allow for junk foods, deplete you instead of nourish you. Follow these simple instructions and your pregnancy will go much easier and your child will be much healthier.

If you add 50 or 60 calories a week, as long as you supplement with Lemmon's Oil and Multi-Nutrient Formula, you will remain devoid of those cravings, remain fit, not fat, give birth like you rehearsed it a million times already and you will lose the additional weight you gain much easier than anyone else you know. Many women report the delivery process being such a breeze that they almost forgot they even had a baby that day.

If you are starting the diet the day you know you're pregnant and you're currently eating 1500 calories a day, try the following:

Week 1, continue having 1600 calories a day...

Week 2 have 1650 calories a day.

Week 3: 1700. Week 4: 1750. Week 5: 1800. Week 6: 1850. Week 7: 1900. Week 8: 1950. Week 9: 2000. Week 10: 2050. Week 11: 2100. Week 12: 2150. Week 13: 2200. Week 14: 2250. Week 15: 2300. Week 16: 2350.

Week 17: 2400. Week 18: 2450. Week 19: 2500. Week 20: 2550. Week 21: 2600. Week 22: 2650. Week 23: 2700. Week 24: 2750. Week 25: 2800. Week 26: 2850. Week 27: 2900. Week 28: 2950. Week 29: 3000.

AND Week 30, have 3050 calories a day.

Although there are 6 to 9 more weeks left until your child arrives, I cannot recommend that you eat more than this each day. I personally haven't met a woman needing more than 3000 calories a day yet. Who knows, you may be the first, but eat clean. Eat very, very clean. Your baby can get clogged arteries just like you can… After child birth, trim your hips, thighs, belly and butt by cutting back 200 calories a week until you are back down to a couple hundred more calories than you started the diet on. Say if you began at 1600, drop 200 calories a week until you're back down to 1800. Do not drop your calories faster than that, it'll startle your metabolism. Besides, you're healing and nursing.

However, once you're down to that "1800" level, stay there until you visibly tighten up. You will, but be patient and do not make a move without your physician's guidance. For those of you not pregnant, I want you to continue to monitor your waist measurement each week. DON'T SUCK IT IN and pretend you've made progress. Deal with reality. It's so much more exciting. And keep track of everything that you are experiencing on our Know How log sheets. I am not saying everyone 'should' agree with keeping a log book. When things are not working for me, I look at my notes. When things are working well for me, I again look at my notes to see what I am doing correctly. I personally like to know what barriers I have hurdled or what ones I need to approach differently.

You may or may not notice change for the better at first or you may feel like you are definitely heading toward a turn for the worse. If this is the case, re-evaluate your starting point.

You probably over estimated your original caloric intake or lied to yourself about how many inches you had to lose to begin with. Or, if you're right on the money, you may only need to be a little more patient. Wait another week to add more calories. That's not too much to ask is it? Your metabolism is still sluggish, but you will be fine. All that abuse you put your body through over the years takes a little time to reverse folks. Sure you may feel behind schedule and possibly discouraged, but you are learning more and more about your body at the same time. Like all things in life, it's a process. It's also something you should have paid closer attention to long ago. So remain patient and move forward at the you're rate your body allows and learn a little about yourselves along the way.

Men should add 40 to 50 calories a week and women only around 20 to 25. Don't bother trying to divide those calories up to add them a little bit to each meal. 5 or 10 calories here and there are too hard to trace. Do it this way instead:

Week One: Follow your estimated calorie levels.
Week Two: Add calories to your Breakfast.
Week Three: Add calories to your Lunch.
Week Four: Add calories to your Brunch.
Week Five: Add calories to your Mid Day Snack.
Week Six: Add calories to your Dinner.
Week Seven: Add calories to your Breakfast again.
Week Eight: Add calories to your Lunch again.
Week Nine: Add calories to your Brunch again.
Week Ten: Add calories to your Mid Day Snack.
Week Eleven: Add the calories to your Dinner again.
Week Twelve: Add calories to your Breakfast.
Week Thirteen: Add calories to Lunch one more time.

For the majority of you, this is all you'll need and there won't be a worry in the world. The only reason there may be is if you think your muscle mass is more than it really is to begin with.

If you are worried about what results to expect and think progress is based on particular body structures, STOP. Don't worry. You're not that different than anybody else. It's simple. An 'ecto' morph is a thin person. A 'meso' morph is a medium sized person. An 'endo' morph is a bigger person. None of this really matters though in regards to your progress or what routine to follow unless you want to have a boring conversation with someone else trying to sound smart. I am explaining it only because many before you have enquired about it. Using Greek terms to describe things like body composition and musculature is silly in the scope of simply tossing the correct foods down your neck for a change. All you need to know about losing fat and building muscle you've already read today.

To build muscle, you must drop body fat. To drop body fat you must build muscle. To accomplish this, some need to eat less. Some need to eat more. Knowing much of anything else really doesn't matter. Only your eating habits matter. When you get someone who is underweight on this diet, they are automatically going to GAIN muscular weight without getting fat. If you get somebody who is currently overweight on this diet, that person is going to start losing weight in the form of fat. It's the natural process the body follows when properly nourished. But you MUST eat enough...

I was told at age 16 by our family physician when I was wanting to gain weight that I was an 'ecto' morph and would never weigh more than 150 pounds. That's funny because when I was born, I was 10 pounds and the doctor said I was an 'endo' morph who was going to be a beast in size by adulthood. I weighed 108 when I was 16. I weighed 150 a little while later at age 17. Eventually I was 274 and drug free when I took up bodybuilding. So I hardly think your current bone size makes much of a difference. Only your diet does. And what percentage of proteins, fats and carbs are best? For now, as long as you get more protein than fat and your carbs are clean, it doesn't matter.

FALLING OFF THE WAGON AND CHEAT DAYS

What about cheating (as in mixing your foods INCORRECTLY)? People don't realize that when they are about to cheat on something that it has a healthier alternative. The desire to cheat should be read as a specific signal from the body as something other than the obvious. Some people reach for potato chips, others reach for candy. One craving is for sugar, and the other is not for salt but for minerals. Some crave steak. That's a protein craving.

Each and every one of us has different cravings and each of them are different signals. If you crave proteins, have something healthy with protein in it. If you crave salty food, get some green vegetables in you. If you crave sugar, you are really in need of essential fats. Foot the bill and you'll fit into your favorite clothing in no time. Revert back to your old eating habits and I cannot be held accountable. As long as you can determine whether what you want is a fat, a protein or a carbohydrate food, you can literally continue to eat anything and scare that craving away.

With the exception of what you already know is bad for you, practically anything is allowed. If you want to have something you can't avoid mixing incorrectly (even though there are sugar or fat free versions available of anything you could possibly imagine these days) do so at only that one meal (IF you need to do that at all). Actually, I insist you cheat every now and then on whatever it is you may want. It will teach you a lesson you wouldn't learn otherwise. I feel like a sloppy pig when I eat badly. I get gas that scares the neighbors. I get headaches and am a bear to be around. But it's your choice. Live how you want. If you do cheat, even by accident or in the event of an emergency because it was between deciding to starve or…

Whether to eat anything you can get your hands on (which is rare), pull your car over, buy a burger at a fast food joint, throw the bun out or run to the grocery store for fruit, nuts or cold cuts.

In the future, always have food and water packed to travel with you nearby. And when you have something you probably shouldn't, don't go overboard. Try to stay within your calorie range for the meal anyhow and resume the program on schedule like nothing ever happened (forget that you ever cheated) afterwards. Whatever the case is, do not skip the next meal just because you feel guilty. Take complete responsibility for the consequences of your own actions, learn from them and climb back on the wagon. Blowing one meal is no big deal.

Skipping a meal is! If you cheat, you set yourself back a day. If you skip a meal, you set yourself back another day. When eating out you cannot control the serving sizes you receive, so remember that you are not obligated to clean your plate. Ask for a doggy bag. If you aren't sure what to get when out with friends, I find ordering only meat and steamed veggies with a side salad but no croutons always works. If you ask for a little butter and Caesar's dressing to dip your fork in to take bites from your salad, no one will think you're eating weird.

I avoid anything Alfredo, battered, breaded, creamed, crisped, or deep-fried like they contain a plague because Lord only knows what all is in these dishes. Seize control of your dining decisions. Let nothing and no one stand in your way. I know some diets are much more lenient. The reason those other programs advocate cheating or even eating more foods on weekends is because those diets want you to take longer to reach your goals. Seriously. If you cheat, you get fat. You get fat, you go out and buy more of their products and stay on their systems even longer. It's actually brilliant from a marketing perspective.

However, this only leads to personal failure, low self-esteem, a lot of wasted time, frustration, enclosure, dead ends, harbored emotions, and a fat, sloppy looking body. Do you know why people you admire most never seem to fail? They don't quit. The definition of "failure" is "quitter." Talent is not their secret.

There are, granted, many keys to success and talent may be one of them, BUT this "know how" is an "education" that leads towards "understanding." Your ability to understand is based upon your desire to become educated. Desire IS based upon determination. Determined people are disciplined through education to succeed by the best means possible. However, successful people CREATE their talent. If you self-discipline yourself, you will not be intimidated by anything between you and the desire of reaching your goals. That takes something beyond talent and education. It takes patience. Sure, you'll make some mistakes and there will be roadblocks but pay attention to them. Roadblocks and mistakes are merely opportunities from which you can gain greater knowledge. Higher learning. Better understanding. Everything you do in life is a chance to become more talented. You will learn things you need to succeed instead of fail if you walk patiently forward in life. Things I can't personally teach you are gained from experience.

This particular experience is RE-CREATION-AL, as in FUN-creating, or creating fun and it is not so much 'work' after all. You'll like this. But some of you will quit anyways. You will not only fail, but learn, therefore understand, succeed or solve ANYTHING for yourself. Nor will you gain talent. Worrying about this only puts off solving the problem, moving forward. There has never been a single thing solved through worry. Worrying, is in fact, so NOT right, it's totally WRONG. I understand that occasionally people aren't trying to be stubborn, or hard headed. They sincerely don't understand all that is laid before them. Well, let me be the first to tell you something else... YOU DO NOT NEED TO UNDERSTAND MOST THINGS IN LIFE TO PUT THE EFFORT INTO MOVING FORWARD.

So welcome back to REALITY. Put your issues and everything else negative behind you. It's time to move forward. "If you think you can, or if you think you can't, you are absolutely right." Believe in yourself. Don't drive yourself nuts thinking life's little pleasures are gone for good and this isn't going to be any fun.

How long is the wait? Well, first, get to your goal. Why would you want to do anything that prevents you from getting to where you want to be safely without any headaches?

Once you succeed, say when you can see your stomach muscles, you can cheat, but only on specific days. How old are you? At the time I wrote this I was 30, so I cheat only once every 30 days. Are you 53? You could realistically cheat every 53 days then. The older you get, the more sensitive your digestive system becomes (like sewage pipes, they go bad in time, only yours can't be replaced, so keep them healthy). A 16 year old could cheat almost every other week. Allowing for more than that is exactly why you haven't gotten where you have liked or struggled to get there if you have. I know some diets are much more lenient.

The reason some diets advocate cheating is because it sets you back and you'll stay on their program longer and longer buying more and more of their products as you go . You really don't have to cheat at all if you do not want to. But go ahead, it's OK. I said you could. If you are going crazy, once a week sounds fine if you are in good shape already, but I just want you to take care of YOURSELF. If you crave carbs, have protein. If you crave salts, have carbs, but only have good clean sources of these foods if you want to remain on track. Once a month I used to get a slice of peanut butter pie from the Hard Rock Café. They no longer serve it. I went 2 years until I had that pie again but it was at the Winking Lizard in Independence, Ohio. That is the only thing I can remember wanting in years. I still want a piece, but I do not CRAVE ONE and THAT is the difference…

Media hype may tell us Jennifer Lopez's big butt is supposed to be attractive. She's pretty, but that butt isn't. Society also tells us music groups that do not write their own songs are talented. Kids believe they do. Next week they will tell us something different. Step away from it all. Do not use what 'everyone says' or 'knows' as a gauge for what YOU should believe in or do.

DIFFERENCES BETWEEN PROGRAMS

This program is based upon what works with, as opposed to against, the human body's natural mechanisms. After working with thousands of folks ranging from the dis-eased, obese and anorexic to clients with close to 300 pounds of lean muscular body mass, I am certain I have found what REALLY WORKS. Not only that, but I know how to keep it working. Without the same hands on experience such as I have put into this, without the same passion I have put into this product, ANY-BODY ELSE'S theory, while possibly an educated guess, is still only A GUESS.

That is why many of my competitors have failed you. No passion. Not as much experience as you'd think. Most of them are nothing more than mouthpieces and spokespeople. I have worked with and spoke with most of the leaders in the bodybuilding and fitness industry. I have literally gathered information from all around the globe and it has always come down to being the same old story. Most people achieve their goals by accident. Hard work and perseverance are taken into consideration, but if you ask people what works, they are still looking for it. It's amazing.

This chapter was written to address the readers who feel they know something I do not. I never claimed to know everything there is to know but what I do know has left quite a few people more than envious. So this goes out to those of you wanting to say I am wrong in one way or another even though you're not sure why. Hey, I made sure all the facts are right here for you to review. I could go on for hours giving you more to go on and yet no matter how much sense I make, there are always going to be those of you saying they already 'know' or believe something else other than I do. I am not sure how that makes me incorrect. Well, do your own research. Examine a few basic medical texts. Tell me another time who is right on the money. Or at least send me a copy of your own book while you're at it.

Besides, if 'everybody knows' this or that, why are so many people still out of shape while following 'this' or 'that' then? On this program, I have seen muscle weight increase from 180 to 240 pounds. I have seen others go from 150 to 210 pounds. I have seen the diabetic decrease their insulin dosages. I have seen the hypoglycemic lead a normal life.

I have seen the elderly tone up. I have seen chubby kids become fit young men and women. All it took was changing their eating habits. What you have learned getting this far through the book should explain why what you have been doing up until now may or may not "work" after all. You should also now have a pretty sound idea why some of what you are doing will NEVER work. But then again, I too realize there remains a small percentage of you reading this book simply out of curiosity whom continue to feel that unless you follow a lower fat diet, the Zone diet, the Atkins diet, food combining, 40-30-30 nutrition, the Protein Power plan or a vegetarian routine, you can't succeed. I must have failed in saving you.

Most diet plans have just enough truth to them and contain enough commonly known facts to make them appear credible or at least difficult to totally discredit. That's what sucks you in only to fail again. And just in case you believe that you need to study your blood type at a school of higher learning to assure results, I suggest having your blood tested immediately. Certainly. And keep the results. Do this so you can see for yourself and show everyone you know how much nonsense you used to believe. Have the plasma, erthrocytes, leucocytes and platelets all examined.

That's all four major constituents of your blood. Just ask for a "CBC" test. Go back and have it all done again in 6 weeks too. See if it mattered one bit what your blood type was when you started after all. You owe yourself that much. Remember, you can actually follow any of the competitive diet plans using the food separation advice I have given you in the 12 Food Groups.

Try me for 6 weeks. You might finally get somewhere. I hope you were able to grasp at least that much already. And no, I haven't forgotten about those of you who are Body for Life cultists nor the high fat dieters in our congregation today (I am joking about the religious over tone)...

I haven't forgotten any of you. I certainly haven't forgotten the fitness pros and doctors you revere either. Just understand, only a fourth of medical schools OFFER nutrition to their students and only 1 in 4 of those actually TAKE the course. We're not talking about requiring the credit hours to get into medical school or offering it as a secondary degree here. We are talking about these people that you put your faith into only having at the most 12 credit hours, and sometimes LESS in nutritional education. And you are learning more today than most fitness professionals have in all the years they have worked in or around the industry. I am not condemning the medical or fitness fields but I do insist you take control of things on your own for a change.

Your health practitioner may like to remind you that they know best because they are physicians or your trainer might think they know best too but that's often only to bully you from asking questions. If being in the medical profession was all it took to be so smart, why aren't ALL doctors in agreement? Because they are in different branches of their field? Ok, why then do so many doctors in the same fields of medicine disagree? Because they all know so very little about nutrition.

They weren't taught it in school and they do not practice it at home. Titles mean nothing. It's TOO EASY for them to simply brush off someone telling the truth when it saves their butts for having misguided you all the while anyhow. Even worse, dieticians and nutritionists these days are being pumped out of schools like robots or puppets on assembly lines too. They are taught their ABC's about certain areas of their field then set free to dispense their newfound knowledge upon the world.

Sadly enough, it's painstakingly obvious so few of these people conduct actual research outside of what is required of them to graduate. They are parrots for their cult. Why do I say that? I can't help but question why so many nutritionists, dieticians and other food industry professionals are so sickly looking, fat, and out of shape if they know something more than what I am telling you. It's hard to find a registered dietician or a certified nutritionist who look their part. If you find one, that's the exception, not the rule. Trainers too are limited in knowledge as well because for some reason, their certifications only cover the basics as set forth by the AMA (American Medical Association) and they usually learn all they are required in an 8 hour weekend course taken at their gyms.

Back to square one. I hope you realize that just because someone has a certification or a degree in this or that, it doesn't make them qualified to dispense advice on these subjects I have covered. I cringe at the thought some trainers are employed at all. And, guess what else? If you believe what you read in the magazines or hear in the news about your eating, you've been misled again. By who? By those doctors, nutritionists and trainers who've now listened to those handling the marketing of your favorite diet or fitness products.

These people only get away with it because they know you're desperate enough to believe and willing to try anything to see results! All I am saying is that the fitness industry is hardly run by professionals with any real qualifications. It is run by people trying to make a buck or two off of people like you, hoping you believe everything you are marketed. So if you believe Bill Phillips or Metrx are 100% honest, you probably believe Britney Spears sings her own songs in concert or the Backstreet Boys created their own dance moves. It doesn't matter if someone has a best seller either. They will come and go. Pet Rocks were best sellers at one time too my friend.

Tip: For those of you investing in CLA and HMB at your local health food store, consider this, CLA and HMB can be obtained for pennies on the dollar by eating 2 tablespoons of raw cream and just 1 tablespoon of real butter a day. All cream and dairy fat contains CLA (a fat that regulates hormones). It's 0.1 to 0.5% of the total fat. If nothing else, that beats paying the $40 a bottle at a health food store for CLA supplements.

Yeah, yeah, surprise, surprise, you thought the people in the white lab coats, the ones you read about in the magazines or saw on late night TV were the prophets of our times and had all your answers. Wake up. They are for the most part borderline clueless, lying through their teeth to cover their tracks or just trying to sell you something. You've all been misled. I put this system together to serve myself. I didn't write it for you or anyone else in the beginning. In fact, I hid what I knew for a long time.

It wasn't until I saw what the industry was doing to us each passing generation that I started giving my advice away. I didn't even charge a dime for it either until I realized I wouldn't be able to put solid effort into actually serving people unless turned it into something I could do full time. I have come a long way since then but I do not flaunt flashy cars, brag of having several homes, or wearing expensive jewelry. You're more likely to catch me in a t-shirt, blue jeans, baseball hat and tennis shoes at a $4.99 buffet than you are seeing me pay $50 for a fancy meal dressed up somewhere needing reservations.

In fact, I give my lectures in jeans and a t-shirt most of the time. I am no different and no better than anyone else, unless of course, you are counting my desire, passion and sincerity towards what I do. I love to meet new people and am not greedy about setting consultation fees. I will often hook up with out-of-town clients for the price of a buffet, so do not think for a second I am wearing different pants than you do.

Since this all began, my clientele has now extended and grown to thousands of people. Each one of you have wonderful stories to tell. Every walk of life from soap opera stars, television personalities, Playboy Playmates and yes, everyday people like ourselves who do all sorts of things from all across the globe have been on this program. I have seen people experience a tremendous amount of fat loss on the exact same program used by those that were looking to gain weight. And I mean obscene amounts of weight gain like going from 160 to 225 in six months (while not gaining even a single ounce of fat) on the same routine another person used to go from 450 "oh my God, that's fat" pounds down to 225 pounds and looking like they were never obese to begin with.

I know, you want to know more about the celebrities I work with. What did they do? The same program. Well why don't I list more of them then? Catch 22. From 1996 to 2000 I had the winners of virtually every single professional female fitness event in the World come film for my workout videos, on my program or have some sort on involvement with me. Mr. America Lee Apperson was in one video, Danny Weigand, a USA Champion, was in another. I could go on and on. You've probably seen my site already.

But why didn't I use more famous people if I work with celebrities? Hmmm. Many current and former clients are rock stars, politicians, super models, actors, professional athletes, fitness stars and bodybuilders and are not listed or discussed because for one, most are under endorsement contracts that do not allow them to 'advocate' me and two, because others like their privacy. No one wants the world to know they put on a few pounds, you know ^? And since I do not pay the others for their testimonials, it only makes sense they look elsewhere for funding their careers. Maybe one day I will consider sponsoring some of my clients but it is not within my budget to pay the latest home run king or academy award-winning director for their public support.

I cannot compete with soft drink or athletic wear manufacturers. Don't ask me about the bigger named supplement companies either. Body For Life or any of the other 'transformation' programs you can count on one hand are designed entirely on getting you to buy $300 a month worth of products from the ring-leaders of the system. Look at whomever is sponsoring the contests. It's someone selling a product line. Never fails. Sure, some say you do not 'have' to use 'their' products but you better if you expect to get recognized! I remember when Body For Life used to require receipts for your supplement purchases to even enter. Most of the time, if there is that sort of hype surrounding a specific supplement line, like Met-rx, that means they are trying to make big money, sure, but that's also a clue that there is something they aren't telling us too. Meaning it's not what we think it is. Why would you need so much hype if you had the magic product? Wouldn't word spread on it's own? Why would you need to promise someone fame if they succeed? Because that's what it is all about.

People want recognized and told they are as good or better than the next guy. Know right now that you already are. Besides, if Met-Rx were really a 'metabolic prescription' which is what the medical term 'met-rx' stands for, why not call it that? Because it isn't one. And so you know, it costs most companies only 10 cents to fill a packet full of meal replacement powder while they turn around and sell it for $4 each at the health food store. I remember when it used to be that if you bought health food, it may have been expensive, you at least got what you paid for. Go out and read whatever you like. Learn. Explore.

After reading this book, you will spot the hidden agendas of others right off the bat. I am sincere when I say I am devoted to human health and drug-free physique enhancement (with or without the desire or genetics for bodybuilding, weightlifting, modeling, or athletics). I have put everything I own including my heart and soul into formulating this program and our two prized supplements.

This book and those two products supply us with 100% of the essential nutrients science tells us we need just to survive. Nothing more is necessary. I do not care who's program you follow, if you apply at least that much, your routine will work better.

I do not ask you to buy creatine, glutamine, meal replacements, or any other mumbo jumbo from me. In fact, if you do not want to try my products at all, you still need those 100 nutrients. Creatine is not technically part of your food. It is something that exists in your body but it isn't necessarily an important food nutrient. The body makes it's own out of other nutrients that are in the foods that contain it. Ironic, I know. But that's how it is. You see, all those guys taking extra with their food are actually confusing the process and preventing the body from absorbing that and other nutrients.

If you take the creatine between meals, or AFTER a carbohydrate meal and you have over 200 pounds of lean mass, it should work. I do not mean taking it directly after. I mean using it between a carb and a protein meal. So if you are going to have carbs at 8:00 a.m. in the morning and protein at 10:30 a.m. then 9:30 a.m. which is halfway between finishing your last meal. Hypothetically that is 8:30 a.m. Mix the creatine in just a little bit of water, swish it in your mouth, hold it there a few seconds and then finally suck it down. Creatine is most efficiently loaded when taken in the presence of elevated blood sugar levels like after a carb meal.

If you take it with your food, or sugar, that's not going to be enough time for the body to raise that blood sugar. You'll get nowhere. And with or without my supplements, you also need to put what else I have taught you into action just to see for yourself if I am right. Don't listen to anyone else. If I am showing you a side of myself you didn't expect to see, good. Let's get it all out in the open. It isn't a matter of "Why is this guy talking to me like this?"

It is more of the question of "Why am I not listening to him yet?" I may not bend on my beliefs but that's because bending is what got you here. It's time for change and being nice hasn't convinced you to do so.

I had the same fears about change as you do at one point. Sure, I have been working with people off and on since 1986, starting off in Ohio where I was born and eventually moving to North and South Carolina then Los Angeles and Las Vegas. But I wasn't always sure of what I was doing either. Even when I was considering a career in orthopedic surgery, I knew that something was missing from the 'wholistic health' portrait the medical world painted.

I wanted to follow a different path. I didn't know what needed changed, but something did. Oh trust me, I have seen, heard, tried and experienced so much since I started weight lifting just to gain a few pounds as a teenager. Back then I wanted to eat right, whatever that meant, but had little guidance. I remember coming home and having bacon, cheese and breaded fish sandwiches before my workouts thinking it was good in providing me protein. The last diet that I remember being on, that really catapulted my quest for the correct eating plan, was a low fat, low carbohydrate diet I was supposed to be on for 4 days followed by a low fat, high carbohydrate diet for 4 more days.

It rotated back and forth between the two alternatives again and again for some reason. What stumped me, after feeling myself go from flat to fat week after week, was why other people would continue to do this to themselves. Fit to fat, fit to fat, blah. Nonsense. I figured this whole low carb thing followed by the high carb loading phase 'had' to have some sort of a happy medium where one could simply be eating right, not yo-yoing around. Couldn't it? Why couldn't it work if you had just 'enough' carbs? Not too little but not too much, 'just' enough...

Something just didn't add up to me still. In fact, my friend Dr. Dave Williams from Las Vegas, Nevada will remember our conversations on what I called dietary 'happy' balances. We agreed it had nothing to do with 'all things' in moderation. No, because people use that term as an excuse to eat cake and candy not essential fats and clean food. I just didn't know back then how to explain it. I only knew how to accomplish it. So like with that last diet I followed, I noticed that if I ate real lean, say mostly tuna and chicken and vegetables during the week, I would definitely get leaner but I also looked 'flat' because of not eating any starchy carbs. My muscles were depleted and empty.

I actually found myself dreaming at night about cheating on my diet in my sleep. I know I wasn't the only one suffering through such a thing but I also knew that I wasn't having these nightmares when my carb intake was higher. I was being starved. So, I evaluated the routine. After 4 days of carbs, I was sick of feeling fat. Instead of having 4 days of low carbohydrate intake followed by 4 days of loading up on carbohydrates, I had a different plan. We decided we would eat high protein and veggies during the work week, then Friday night we would let loose.

I worked and studied during the week. He worked too. Like every other student and 9 to 5'er, I wanted to enjoy myself those 2 days of the week and relax. So that's what we did. As soon as the boss sent us home on Fridays, we ordered pizza. I liked mine low fat vegetarian style. Saturday morning would be our breakfast buffet (of eggs, sausage, bacon, and cottage cheese) at the local diner. Saturday afternoon was the steak house buffet (carbs mostly like rice, pasta, potatoes and salad). And Saturday evenings we split a case of beer. Hey, just being honest. I drank beer. I also said I knew I needed a change and here I am evaluating exactly what that was...

Sunday's lunch (without fail) was always six 99-cent double cheese burgers (I would throw out the buns) but all the other meals were typical snacks like yogurt, chicken breasts, fish, etc. It didn't take a genius to determine if you eat this much on weekends, you must be REALLY depleted from what you weren't eating during the rest of the week! My body was craving things and I was literally sucking them down. By the end of each weekend, no matter how well I ate, and I did eat clean most of the time, I still felt bloated.

It wasn't just that I was loading up on both carbohydrates and protein, my metabolism had slowed during the week and 48 hours wasn't enough time to speed it back up. I knew I was eating good food, despite the beer, but I was still depleting myself and feeling like I fattened up all over again. And I was getting sick from colds or flus too it seemed every single month. Enough was enough. I stopped. By the end of the next six month period of simply eating the same foods and separating them from one another, like having carbs at only a couple meals a day instead of 14 of them over a weekend, I went from 195 puffy pounds to 215 lean pounds.

I hadn't changed my overall calorie intake at all either. I had found a happy medium instead. I quit the 2000 calories a day for 5 days followed by 6000 calories a day for 2 days and added it all up to average 3200 calories a day. That's what I ate. 3200 calories a day. Those depletion diets always said you should eat your carbs without fat or protein if you want them to load properly without bloating yet they had you eating carbs, fats and proteins together to gain weight. I didn't understand how one was supposed to lean you, but the other fattened you. And why would you want that?

I realized that I was feeling better eating carbs alone at some meals and only proteins and fats at others, but not so good when I cheated and had ate all three together, but how could I have better results than ever before with so little effort?

I wondered why someone else hadn't recognized this before. I became a walking testimony that the stomach has no means by which to digest commercially processed foods or separate poorly combined foods. I was living proof and that's all there was to it. Wow, it was like yesterday. Then again...

Sometimes I feel like I just woke up one day training athletes and celebrities in Vegas and California and yet it's actually been so long ago that I figured all of this out. What began as a courtesy of putting friends and patients on eating plans that I myself had been following has turned into something so much more. Food Separation was at first just something that I felt was natural.

I was in fantastic shape year round, my health was returning from where I really didn't want it to be and I was only exercising twice a week. So I knew I was on to something. Results are based upon nutritional habits, not my efforts in the gym.

Still, for a while there, many unanswered questions like 'why does it work' were being asked by my clients and I wanted to be able to provide them answers. They do not teach nutrition in medical school folks. So I was on my own if I wanted solutions or answers. This is what led to my research, studying, reading, and eventually writing this very book. If I hadn't wanted you to succeed in life as much as I have, I wouldn't have stepped down from the medical field and we wouldn't have Don Lemmon's Know How. Right now, all I ask is that you willingly climb out of the hole you dug for yourself and get in gear.

If that bothers you, it still isn't me that you are mad at. I understand you may have dealt with a few fitness industry nightmares in the past and are afraid of failing again. I feel for you but I am not allowing you to use what's happened to you in the past as a crutch any longer. You can and I do expect you to depend upon me. So co-operate with me here and I will co-operate with you.

I know this is all very new to you too like it is to everyone else reading my book for the first time and you are simply trying to sort it all out in your head before deciding to start. Problem is, trying to apply logic to what you know so little about wastes all the time you could have spent trying something new. By the time you got around to knowing more about what I suggest, you could already have washboard abs if you'll only start today. It took me YEARS to straighten all this out and you're just wasting away whether we agree or not. No one wants to feel like they didn't 'know' something. But how could you of known something unless you were taught it or discovered it? That's what I am here for. Let's promise one another not to quit just because where we disagree isn't on whether what I do works, but whether you understand WHY it works. We all know how to operate a car but you won't catch many of us designing one anytime soon. All I know is that if I take care of my car, sometimes see a mechanic and stick a key in the ignition, my vehicle will last me a long time and run properly.

One sure fire reason our approach works is not only because proper mixtures of food complements your digestive system so well but it's this fact that ALLOWS you to eat more often and have more food. More food means more nourishment! It's not a ticket to over eat, but your old 1000 calorie a day diets are now a thing of the past with us. In fact, many women start this program at 1800 calories a day and men start somewhere near 3000 calories a day. Can you imagine? Eating like royalty while experiencing results you never before dreamed possible! By looking before you leap, thinking a little before putting something in your mouth from now on, you can do exactly that! NO MATTER THE PROGRAM! I am sure whatever program it was you were on last probably did in fact work for a while. If you toy with your calories a bit, eat a little cleaner or better than you did before, maybe stopped having fat with carbs or vice versa and started to exercise a little more, most all programs do work for a while.

Anything can show minimal results and it's those results that pull us in thinking that it's the only thing that will work for you. Despite those minimal results that had you swearing by your program for however long you were on it, you're still here today for a reason and I have a handful of questions to ask.

1) When did that last diet finally QUIT working for you?
2) Why all of a sudden did it fail at all?
3) Did that diet leave you with unattractive loose fitting skin or more than 10 pounds of fat left to lose?
4) How do you get yourself out of such a rut?
5) Can you see your abdominal muscles at all?
6) Was anything you followed even close to being a practical program you could follow forever?
7) Were their lifestyle limitations?
8) What kind of shape was the author in?
9) Did the author have plastic surgery or take drugs?
10) Are you paying more for your supplements than you are for food each month?

You now know by alternating carbohydrate and fat/protein meals (which yes, somewhat lowers your overall intake of carbohydrates and is a combination of both low fat vegetarian dieting and low carbohydrate meat eating), you can work out the glitches of any program you have ever tried before or are currently following. If you have been eating a low-fat diet, separate your proteins and carbohydrates and add a couple low carbohydrate meals to your daily schedule. If you have been eating a low carbohydrate diet, no problem!

Have some more fibrous greens and add a couple low fat 'no meat' meals to your daily schedule. If you have been mixing proteins, fats and carbohydrates on a diet that leaves you eating in a zone of 30% proteins, 30% fats and 40% carbohydrates, all you have to do is to place the carbohydrates you eat in meals separate from the proteins and fats.

If you are on a physique transformation plan that recommends eating 40/40/20 at all your meals, again, begin food separation and try pouring all those powdered meal replacements down the drain. That alone will make all the difference.

Vegetarians, do not eat tofu with starches and add some organic cottage cheese or farm fresh eggs to your program. It's not so much to ask. You wouldn't be here either if what you were doing was fulfilling you. Don't get mad at me for saying it. You know it's true. This book is nothing more than a compilation put together by myself reflecting my years of effort as a collection of information from different readings, findings, communications, etc, etc, and personal notes based upon the needs and results obtained or required from thousands of people, but no single reference is afforded a lengthy quotation that already hasn't been credited. I have come to believe either you KNOW HOW to do what you do or you DO NOT.

If you go to a doctor, a nutritionist, a dietician, a fitness expert , health food store employee or a personal trainer, let alone a supposedly professional athlete and they have a pot belly, saggy skin, double chins, blotchy flesh or look like they haven't touched a weight in decades, do you really think they have any clue whatsoever about what sort of advice you need to make yourself fit? They aren't fooling me one bit.

You read about out of shape diet gurus, you see their pictures, we run into overweight fitness experts at conventions, physicians who supposedly discovered fat loss secrets but none of these people look like the models advertising their work....

When will America catch on? Who really wants to look like a bodybuilder? Bodybuilders. But who wants to look like these people who authored the biggest diet fads this century? Not me!

And neither should you!

CARBOHYDRATES AS ENERGY

The hesitation people actually have with food separation is ironically due to their thinking this is a low carbohydrate plan believe it or not. Yeah, of all things. Because I only suggest 2 carb meals a day, people think this is a low carb plan. They think they will tire out with only two carb meals, especially during a workout. There are two types of exercise. One is aerobic or 'cardiovascular' exercise, and the other is 'anaerobic' weight (resistance) training. As far as nutrition goes, there isn't much of a difference. Aerobic athletes do tend to require an extra carb meal on marathon days but they could also use an extra protein meal. Competitive weight lifters or bodybuilders also require an extra carb meal after their training sessions, but they too, like anyone else, require only 2 carb meals on off days. Plan your schedule accordingly but I do not care who you are, track athletes, or the general fitness folks, we are all alike in one way and that is you require 4 protein and 2 carb meals a day typically.

First of all, the misconception that you must receive all your energy via glycogen, glucose and carbohydrates is incorrect. And despite it being considered the most logical idea to reduce carbs to lose fat, it is another myth that you need to eliminate carbohydrates altogether from your diet in order to burn body fat. All you have to do is 'reduce' them, not eliminate them. Low carbohydrate or 'ketogenic' diets are hazardous. Did you know being in a constant state of ketosis means your body is not adapting correctly to your diet? It is actually a sign that it has begun breaking itself down. Despite the fact that they say the hormones released while on a low carb plan (glucocorticoids and glucagon) mobilize the liver's reserve of glycogen (carbs), so you burn fat, that's not exactly how it works. Keeping the liver low in carbohydrates for efficiency reasons is one thing, but the muscles are the next thing to be burnt and you don't want that to happen. You will fall flat (which always happens once your muscle glycogen is lost).

Anyways, this isn't a low carb diet. I want you to eat carbs twice a day without fail. This is a decrease for some of you and an increase for others. Adjusting your carbohydrate intake slightly either way will not adversely affect you if you also increasing your essential fatty acids. This is because good fats work well with protein. Carbs do not. And while carbs might interfere with other metabolic processes or deplete you of minerals whereas fats do not, you won't be eating that many carbs if you only have them twice a day.

In regards to the idea following other diets that in order to use proteins properly you need to eat them with carbs, having carbs at every meal only makes you carb dependant, and a sugar addict. Sure, you can always do 60 minutes of aerobics twice a day, mix your foods, and stay fairly lean if you eat low fat, but that's like racing your truck uphill with a trailer hitched on the back. Instead you should be driving a much efficient vehicle that runs on better fuel to get the job done easier. Almost any vehicle will get you to the top, but one doesn't force you to work so hard nor wonder if you're ever actually going to make it to the top at all.

I choose the high performance vehicle. Either way, a carbohydrate dependent body is NOT a good thing. The body's attempt to produce most of its energy from carbohydrates is why you cramp and burn during exercise. It is from the buildup of lactic acid that high carb intakes produce. Do you lie awake sleepless at night or get cramps that are almost unbearable? That's from either having too many sugars in your diet or even worse, a lack of the nutrients which prevent the cramping.

If you are getting what you feel is enough nutrition but you still cramp, you may want to look into the type of carbohydrate you ingest or the quality of the products you use. Alcoholics get cramps all the time by the way. Alcohol depletes minerals....

Marketing hype may have you believing you need carbs for their sugars in order to transport your proteins but no matter what this simply isn't true. The body eventually turns everything you eat into one form of sugar or another (and ultimately all sugar gets turned into various forms of alcohol before it is entirely processed) and that includes proteins and fats. Sure, you can argue that you need all three nutrients in lesser or equal values as per the Zone diet but I beg to differ the rationale.

When glucose enters the bloodstream after the digestion of carbohydrates, proteins or fats, insulin eventually gets secreted by the pancreas to utilize them. From there, the next step is going to be either good or bad based upon the nutrients currently available inside of you or what you just ate. If you ate too much carbohydrate food for instance, it cannot and will not be stored as glycogen even if there are sufficient nutrients and enzymes available in the bloodstream to do so. There is only 'so much' room to store all the carbs you eat in your liver or muscles, folks.

The excess causes a depletion of other vital nutrients to get rid of it and either ends up wasted or stored as fat. Either way, YOU lose, but it depends on what condition you have yourself in right now and what you ate with those carbs that make the difference. The excess or unusable carbohydrates are usually transferred into a form of triglycerides before they are stored as body fat. If you ate fat at this meal with those carbs, guess where that goes once the excess carbs are stored as fat? You guessed it. Around your butt and gut. Birds of a feather flock together my friend. Eventually, when there is a need for more energy that the diet doesn't supply, stored glycogen is, yes, converted back into glucose and used by cells or transported through the bloodstream for further conversion and use. But this only happens during exercise or starvation (which is what low carb diets do... They STARVE you). And even if it is during exercise and not because you are starving, once glycogen is depleted, you will not enter into what you think is a fat burning zone. What? Why not?

Well, you see, glycogen is in limited availability when it comes to energy. It can deplete in as little as 10 to 15 minutes under extreme conditions. Ever worked real hard for 10 straight minutes and began shaking? You depleted yourself of glycogen.

Yes, that quickly. And once it's gone, the body demands that it is immediately replaced or what you think is your fat burning zone actually results in muscle degeneration. This doesn't mean you need more carbohydrates during the exercise session. The body doesn't digest and react that quickly even with simple sugars. Carbohydrates, while they are quick energy sources, were not meant to be your primary source of energy. You need dietary fat for that. No? Then why do the experts say glycogen only lasts you about 20 to 30 minutes MAXIMUM during exercise?

Why do physicians say you burn more muscle than fat once it is gone? Because carbs are meant for short bursts of energy and fat is meant for longer-term use. Before we go any further, it is this depletion of glycogen that is PRECISELY why your exercise sessions must be shortened as well. More on that later. Let's continue. We can solve all of your problems by simply eating fat with protein PRIOR to your workouts. In doing this you are signaling to the body that you want it to protect its glycogen because you are giving it something else to burn. Once it runs out of dietary fat, the body will then begin to BURN BODY FAT during the session leaving the protein alone.

What if the preferred energy source to begin with always was fat? Carbs fill the muscle and organs and then protein builds and heals tissues. You see, the body only uses carbs when it runs low on fat to burn. Then once it runs out of carbs, you'll always burn muscle before anything else. The body then goes scavenging for more and more carbs as replacement. Remember this because without proper fat in the diet, once you run low on glycogen, the body breaks protein down for glucose and you'll continually struggle to make progress. IMAGINE THE RESULTS if you take advantage of what I have just said.

I used to have plain tasting pure whey mixed with filtered water, whole cream and ginger before my workouts but I can no longer find a good source of whey from anyone who hasn't 'sold out' and corrupted their product. Since I have gotten fine results on the coffee and cream alone. Then afterwards I have something like a bagel with raisins or another carb. This is a virtually fool proof method that reverses a number of negative mechanisms happening internally that can cause you to feel drained, exhausted, aggravated, fatigued, and etc if you do not do pay attention. Even if you do not understand, you WILL AT LEAST recover faster from your training this way.

And recovery from working out, despite the other stresses of everyday living, is what allows for progress. How is that possible? Well, it is still recommended that you eat carbs separate from your proteins. But once food digests, it enters your bloodstream. This is what elevates your blood sugar levels or the amount of protein available inside of your body. What occurs next is actually a constant lingering of available glucose or amino acids that's still available when you eat one or two of your following meals. This is the reason why we have protein meals before our workouts and save the carbohydrates for afterwards. I know it is the opposite that most experts suggest but protein digests slowly, carbs digest faster.

So if you eat your protein now, in about 2 hours once it has digested, the amino acids from that protein meal will then be just about ready and waiting in your bloodstream to start healing your sore muscles. If you eat carbs at the correct times, like just as soon as the workout is over, then the glucose will enter the system in time to assist the protein to your tissues for recovery. Those same carbs will also still be around for the benefit of your next couple of meals if you eat enough (but not too much mind you). If you eat carbs at the wrong times, like before a workout, you'll end up fat...

Does that make it simple enough to understand? It is what you eat now, that makes food work better for you when you eat again later... That covers your workouts, muscle building, fat burning, etc. But in everyday life, there are still three basic steps in the production of energy whether it comes through fat, protein or carbohydrate metabolism. We know that once any food is eaten it is turned to glucose or sugar and those three steps by which it's done are glycolysis, the citric acid cycle (CAC or Kreb's cycle) and the electron transport chain (ETC).

The net result of the entire production is something called ATP (adenosine tri-phosphate). ATP is the energy source of just about everything we do. It is an organic chemical compound that acts like a converter, controlling the power switches that keeps us alive. ATP is constantly being manufactured, stored, and burned 24 hours a day. Chronic fatigue is one of the most common problems plaguing society today, second only to obesity and a lack of ATP explains why. You see, of the food we eat, almost half of it is supposed to keep our metabolism going. The other half is supposed to provide energy in the form of ATP.

The process of manufacturing ATP is known as oxidative phosphorylation, which is merely the coupling of phosphorus and adenosine. But before we can even begin to worry about this, we need to understand that carbohydrates may not be the best fuel in initiating the phosphorylation process. Glycosis and CAC provide the groundwork for the ETC process. Luckily, Glycolysis can generate the CAC from whatever you eat. However, when it is produced from carbohydrates, because they burn so fast, there is very little raw material left over to perform the third and most crucial step, the building of that electron transport chain (ETC). The first step for fat metabolism however is beta-oxidation, which yields 2 carbon groups for the citric acid cycle to function. An amino acid's (protein molecule's) first step is de-amination, a process where the amino acids are removed from the protein by the liver and the kidneys.

That means fat and protein burn a little slower than carbs do and as we know with all other things, the more careful nature is adhered to, the more efficient you become. Efficiency in this case results in a faster metabolism and more natural energy. No more coffee, no more fatigue.

There's never a lack of energy on this program unless you subject yourself to a lack of sleep, water or food. If you have been following the program but aren't seeing results, then you aren't really 'on' the program. This is precisely why I insist you send your diet to me whenever it changes for re-evaluation. We cannot guarantee you understand everything and are 'on' the 'diet' unless I see with my own two eyes. It's easy to misunderstand something considering my ideas are so radical and new to you. If you send me your daily routine to look at, I will fix everything for you. I promise.

I need to know your name, age, height, weight, and what you eat and drink at all your meals. From there, we will get you on track. As good as this is beginning to sound, simply eating protein and fat together isn't enough if you continue to insist on a low calorie, low carb, and low fat diet. That puts you in a state of serious ketosis (remember, that's muscle burning for energy, and not a good thing). But if sufficient calories are available and enough fat is present, you are safe from muscle wasting. Just how much protein and fat? More of both, especially if you haven't been eating much of either.

Calorie restrictive diets don't work because they remove as much muscle as they do fat and that only makes you look fatter although you look smaller. Muscle is the only engine that burns fat. The more muscle you lose, the less fat you burn. What happens if you haven't had fat in a while? When fat is reintroduced to your diet (even just a little), and carbs are reduced or increased to just two meals a day, most of your energy will almost immediately come from the breakdown of fatty acids.

Initially it will be from the dietary fat but eventually, that unsightly stored body fat will diminish as the cycle continues (which takes from 3 to 7 weeks to fully experience results, you'll know why in a minute) too. The body will not store the fat we suggest you eat. The body only stores fat because either you eat too many carbs, mix your foods incorrectly or you limit fat intake. And we aren't suggesting you eat a lot of fat. We are simply recommending that you add the right fats back into your diet. If you do this and maintain it, the enzymes that break fat down will prevent you from ever becoming overweight again.

Basically, a diet a little higher in fat, activates the lipolytic (fat burning) enzymes in your body and decreases the activity of the lipogenic (fat producing) enzymes. A body which receives too much fat reacts much the same way a body with too many carbohydrates would. You get fat from it. So stick with that 3 to 1 protein to fat gram ratio I recommended in the 12 Food Groups for 4 meals and have carbs at two other meals and you'll be fine.

Now you know, certain other metabolic pathways are blocked if you eat a lot of carbohydrates. The body won't efficiently make energy from glucose, nor use proteins or fats correctly if this happens. This is the theory that conned so many of you to try the Zone. What kept it from working was the same thing that kept anything else from working, the food separation. The result of all those other plans was a continued craving of glucose (sugar) for glycolysis, right? What do you think is going on when we get noticeably drowsy after eating a lot of carbs after you binge? A moderate, or reduced, carb intake prevents drowsiness and binging. Simply reduce or increase your intake to only 2 carb meals a day as soon as possible.

If you go with less or try more right now, depending on what you are used to doing, you will burn out, fatigue, and confuse the other tissues that will then start trying to replace lost carbs… That again means losing muscle.

Subsequently, if you won't heed this advice, hypoglycemia will develop and this stresses not only the adrenal glands but your pancreas. What did we learn today? Carbohydrates are essential to maintaining internal sugar stores, but using them as your primary energy source is like using one lamp to light up an entire house. It doesn't work and your entire system is thrown for a loop. When we run low and we ingest more carbohydrates to replace what is lost, this only 'fuels' us with just 'enough' energy. Forget hypoglycemia or diabetes, hypo-adrenia eventually develops (a state in which your adrenal system becomes stressed trying to pick up the resulting slack you have caused).

This is what I meant when I said you not only get tired, but it's also why you get irritable sometimes after you eat. Two carb meals a day are all you need to stay within the 'too much' or 'too little' ZONE. Just try it. You may not be sure either way what is right. That's why I am here.

To tell you what actually works. It does a lot of good by thinking of carbs as a secondary energy source and EATING more fat than you have in the past. I emphasize this AGAIN, because the body will, under most conditions, take muscle protein and turn it into a form of glucose (via gluconeogenesis) for energy once carbohydrates are exhausted if and essential fatty acids aren't there. Trust me on this. A good analogy to describe ATP use is like comparing the process to an average every day battery. Batteries get overused to a point that all it's capable of producing is unusable fizzles.

Rechargeable batteries that can have energy put back in them can also only perform again if it is replenished first. ATP then is like the higher energy source, the rechargeable battery. ADP is the lesser energy source or a drained battery. ATP becomes ADP if it isn't recharged in time and that's when the body depletes itself looking for something that isn't there to turn itself back into ATP. This is likened to tossing your belongings out of a closet blindly behind you looking for a needle.

Everything goes into disarray and takes quite a while to clean before anything is operating normally again. Let's try to avoid this the best we can.

First thing you should do right now is show this book to your friends if any of them know anything about biochemistry. Get their feedback. Call a professional. See what they say. One thing is for certain, if you soak this all in, your life is about to change. Those around you need to know why and how. Do not keep it a secret you used this program and make sure you can tell them WHY your changes occurred. Of course read the rest of the book first so you can talk the talk after walking the walk.

And by finishing the book first, you'll know why you are experiencing all the negative things that you are these days. If you think the answer lies in an exercise plan, then why hasn't exercise achieved all your goals for you yet? Just keep them in order and once you've gotten through the entire book, send me those questions. Many times my views challenge the supposedly educated and well researched people who figure if they didn't know something already, no one else could either. I am here to help you and I will, despite the fact you are in denial. I am willing to help the most stubborn of you to get on the right path. But remain patient and finish the book first.

This next section is for those of you who require more information as to why fats are so important before you will try them. If you do not add at least one tablespoon of the right (essential) fats a day, NO other supplements you use will fully benefit you NOR will your food digest properly NOR will anything else you do regarding health, work in your favor. If you use lotion for dry skin or your kid uses pimple cream for acne, all they need is some essential fatty acids. Not eating real oil because you are taking only capsules? That is another reason why you're having these problems. Capsules are made by heating oil. Heated oil is dead.

ESSENTIAL VS COMMERCIAL FATS

Without fresh, unheated, raw essential fatty acids, little by little, everything in your entire body eventually fails. No? I haven't met a woman yet who eats a low fat diet that doesn't experience degenerative reproductive system disorders (like not having a period). I haven't met a man yet who eats a low fat diet that doesn't end up with a low sperm or testosterone count. In fact, I had a couple of friends who were smokers and couldn't have a child no matter how hard they tried for the better part of over 10 years. They blamed the smoking. I did too in part because smoking depletes the nutrients essential fats normally try to protect inside of you.

His wife didn't smoke as much, but she did smoke sometimes. And since the husband's family were all chain smokers, she suffered from more second hand smoke than anyone else I had ever known. And to top it off, she was following a low fat diet to 'maintain' her figure. Her hubby was a baker and ate so many pastries that I couldn't even begin to assume how much hydrogenated oil was clogging his veins...

However, even with all this, after just 30 days of taking the essential oil I recommended, she became pregnant. For 10 years, they had nothing. After 4 weeks and 2 days of essential oils, there was a baby on the way. Coincidence? No. She quit taking the supplements after 60 days and lost the baby. Her physician told her that whatever she did to clean up her system over those first 30 days should have been continued. After just 30 days off the supplements, her blood work improved and went back to what it was months before. A baby couldn't form under those conditions. No, these two people weren't fitness competitors, athletes or models. But now that I have your attention, I want to go a bit more in depth so you can understand how essential fatty acids affect all of us. Fats really are the single most important nutrients we require although they only account for 10% of the 100 essential nutrients.

Fat regulates your hormones. Fat also kills your hormones. Fat carries vitamins and minerals to your cells in order to nourish you and if you miss out on taking in enough essential fats on a daily basis, you not only lose out on 10% of what your overall success may be, but you lose out on 33% of what goes on inside of you because the other nutrients and even your organs can't function without them. Over time, this adds up to nothing but trouble.

For example, we mentioned earlier how the liver normally puts excess cholesterol in bile. Well, it is supposed to send it to the gall bladder, which then empties it into the small intestine just below the stomach for excretion. It cannot do this if you're only eating olive oil and cup cakes. It clogs and becomes backed up on a 'normal' diet. You must realize that the removal of excess cholesterol and waste is a natural process that we must accommodate with proper nutrition. If not, we experience elevated cholesterol levels in the blood and disease.

That's right, what I am trying to tell you is that the right kind of fats regulate cholesterol and reverse high blood pressure. Bad fats do not. It's a fact. And essential fats do not make you fat like bad fat does. The body instantly recognizes them as 'good' for you and puts them to use for healing and growth as soon as you ingest them. The difference is that you have to ingest these fats. The body doesn't make essential fats on it's own and they are not contained in things found at the grocery store. Therefore we supplement....

Here is why. There are several kinds of fats, and two are essential (EFA): Omega 3 (n-3 or w3) and Omega 6 (n-6 or w6). All other fats, such as omega 9 (mono-unsaturated), omega 7, and the saturated fats, are non-essential because the body CAN produce these ones quite easily from sugars and starches if need be. Good fats regulate immune and inflammatory responses, lower risk factors for cardiovascular disease, reduce high triglycerides, and even improve your vision. The opposite is true of 'bad' fats. Omega 3's and Omega 6's are good fats.

Omega 9 fats are neutral, so to speak. The important thing to remember is that essential fats must be taken in the right amounts, in proper ratios, just like the suggested RDA percent of vitamins and minerals if we want the best results. Where do we get them?

Usable Omega 6 fats are found in sesame, flax or sunflower seeds and most nuts. Animal meats and many fish sources contain the Omega 6 derivative arachidonic acid (AA) which, while a little different, are just as important as the Omega 6's found in nuts and seeds. Sources of Omega 3's are found in flaxseeds and green leafy vegetables but that's not the same Omega 3 that comes from cold-water fish such as albacore tuna, Atlantic halibut, salmon and shellfish. The problem with fish sources though is that it is almost impossible to ingest enough to supply the fats sufficiently.

This is because of the abundance of essentials needed to meet the body's requirements daily. But we can't give up now! We really do need to get these fats from somewhere. Our brain alone is over 60% fat, and EFA's are vital components to not only the brain but the rest of the nervous system. In fact, if mothers become depleted of EFA's during pregnancy, their children's optimal spine development is limited. As we already discussed, it is common for malnourished women, even those who think they are nourished, to lose their babies. It is well known that EFA's are necessary for every cell's growth from the moment of conception to the day we die.

The common malnourishment we all share began with something that happened in 1900. This is when a different type of fat appeared in our diets. That fat has increased in availability by about 20 times since then. This fat is derived from a particular form of vegetable oil. How can we avoid it? That's hard to say. We are unwittingly eating these bad fats even when we think we are eating 'right.' So, it's no wonder your health has degenerated and you can't get into shape as easy as you would like.

Couple getting bad fats in your health foods with the 'low' fat, 'no' fat, and 'fake' fat diets that have been further depriving people of the good stuff and we've got a lot of work ahead of us if we want to get our health back. So, as of this moment, you need to make the conscious decision to cut out junk food if you want your cholesterol under control. Even 'partially' hydrogenated oils like margarine, although cholesterol free, are bad. Sure, butter (and egg yolks too) contain cholesterol, but they also contain natural fat mobilizing nutrients. When foods are eaten in their own whole food form, they are more than able to metabolize themselves. Margarines do not have this going for them.

Margarines are fake fats made by taking an otherwise 'good' cis-linoleic acid and adding a hydrogen to the double bonds which turns them into un-natural forms of saturated fats in a Frankenstein-ish 'trans' formation. This is done so they last longer on a store shelf and for no other reason. This is unfortunate because you try to eat fat free foods or health food bars and protein powders but only have your blood cholesterol escalate beyond your control. Drop these un-natural fats and foods containing them from your diet and you will have your 'bad' LDL cholesterol levels return to normal quite rapidly (whether or not the genetic tendency runs high in your family).

It isn't genetics which raise your cholesterol. It's your everyday HABITS. The Harvard School of Public Health has warned us for years on the dangers of eating margarines, commercially baked snack goods, and deep fried foods as opposed to using good fats like real butter, extra virgin olive oil (means the olive hasn't fallen from the tree before processing) and Omega 3 fats because it's the processed oils that are making us die slow, painful deaths. Many of those who listened have turned to unrefined flax oil, which is high in omega 3, thinking this will help solve their problem. It doesn't always help.

Using flax oil alone can disrupt the natural balance of things and lead to a shortage of omega 6 fats if you aren't careful. Fats (triglycerides, cholesterols, phospholipids, etc) all produce the precursors to your hormones, tissues and cells. Including the ones for creating either fat loss, muscle growth, normal development or having a baby (from a man or a woman's perspective). But in order to understand why you need such a balance, we need a more in-depth discussion on the GOOD vs. BAD fats. Good fats act as anti-oxidants, anti-inflammatory agents.

They even produce fat burning enzymes. However, you MUST ingest a fat called gamma linolenic acid to activate your 'good' brown fat cells to burn away your ugly 'white' fat cells. Borage oil and primrose oil are good sources of this one. Do you remember me saying that cholesterol is actually a required nutrient? (You get 90 milligrams or so with every 3 ounces of meat you eat.) Well, it regulates your every cell so that actually makes it a good fat. You need it daily. No two ways about it. In fact, under most conditions, two thirds of the cholesterol that is inside of you is produced by the body itself and only a third of it is actually derived from the food you eat.

There are only two explanations for having high or elevated cholesterol. Either you are producing too much of it for some reason (possibly a backed up liver) or you are eating too much of it to begin with (which is only a problem if your body isn't breaking it down). Another good fat is alpha linolenic acid (ALA) which produces the acids that limit the growth of 'bad' hormones, so that's obviously helpful. You can get ALA from walnuts, flax seed, and other cold weather oils. We're not done yet. On top of this, you still need 6 grams per 100 pounds you weigh of linoleic acids. That's about a half tablespoon. Note, I know it's confusing because some acids are spelled or sound nearly the same as others but they are NOT the same type of fats. And remember, 1000 milligrams of any type of fat equals 1 full gram in measure and a gram of fat contains 9 calories each.

This is important because studies throughout the years have shown that 6% of your diet should consist of these essential fatty acids alone. Yet, even more has proven beneficial when it comes to maintaining lower blood fat levels and inhibiting arterial plaque. If you are on a low fat diet, half your fat should be from essentials.

However, if you are on a low carb diet, you will need an extra 4 grams of Omega 3 fish oils (EPA and DHA) combined with a teaspoon of flax seed oil (works synergistically together) to keep your mental acuity straight. DHA (found in both oils) is SO essential that without it, your mind degenerates and you will actually burn brain cells. The reason we mix the two instead of selecting just one is because the Omega 3 fatty acids found in flax seed and walnuts (50% of the flax seed is Omega 3 while walnut oil has only 20%) are totally different sources than Omega 3's from fish. In fact, fish liver oil Omegas are good for night blindness but seed oil Omega 3's are better for renal damage.

This means if you have kidney stones you will not benefit from fish liver oil. But you will from the seed source of oil while very similar, they are different. You must also be careful not to ingest spoiled, over processed, rancid and toxic fat sources. (if it smells like fish, it's spoiled.) Many sources of oils and fish products are. Only fresh oils work. You may as well seal your own coffin taking the oils most outlets supply you. I will tell you where to get your oils in a bit. You now see we need many different kinds of fats. Some are necessary, some we can burn, some we store and some that poison us. Out of all of this, there are really only three that affect us. The differences between the three lie the reason we need to receive these fats in balanced amounts.

Most aging afflictions like heart attacks, strokes, arthritis, and headaches or symptoms such as graying hair, wrinkles, etc... are all related to what we have just discussed so far.

Preventative measures must be taken today to protect you 30 years from now, however, I repeat, simply chugging down some flax seed oil isn't going to do the trick. Every fat we eat, no matter the source, is eventually converted into more specific hormones called prostagladins (PG for short). There are PG1, PG2 and PG3 groups. Groups 1 and 3 are the good hormones, PG2's are the bad guys, at least in the hormone world. PG1 and 3's control blood clots, pressure, swelling, inflammation, and tumors. PG2's do the opposite. PG2's cause dis-ease. PG1's are from fats found in safflower, sunflower, primrose and currant oils. They are Omega 6's. PG1's require several biochemical changes and are dependent upon di-homo-gamma-linolenic acid (DGLA) to butterfly into good hormones.

PG1's are slow and tedious in making this transition process. It takes time to get things right. As for the elderly, this PG1 process is ever important as these particular hormones are the ones which carry calcium and other minerals into your bones and tissues instead of pulling them out like the bad fats do. Get these good fats under control and calcium deposits will become a thing of the past. The other good hormones, the PG3's, are made from fats found in walnut, flax and cold-water fish oils (Omega 3's).

They require but one biochemical change in becoming a hormone from a fat. Reason being, they are equipped with their own "Omega 3 exclusive" EPA (ei-co-sa-pent-ae-no-ic) acid enzyme. It is well known in medical circles that PG3 hormone stimulating fats are fat burning and illness fighting heroes. These fats are good for men looking to raise their testosterone, women to maintain their femininity and even cancer or AIDS patients trying to build their white blood cells. PG2's however, the bad guys, come not only from the fats in red meats, shell fish (neither of these sources are really so bad) but they are ESPECIALLY BAD if they come from hydrogenated oils and fake fats (OH SO VERY BAD).

These fats only require one step instead of several to change into hormones like the PG3's do. Because PG2 fats process the fastest of all the PG's, leaving PG1 and 3's at a biochemical disadvantage, PG2's poison you long before the good guys are around to help you! The Catch 22 occurred when we discovered some of the naturally occurring fats (like stearic acid, which is necessary for a normal metabolism) such as though found in meat and shell fish that breed PG2's. You see, we can have a little PG2 in our system and be safe, but the PG2's that come from oil sources (oils that never spoil) like hydrogenated coconut, palm and baking oils are the problem.

It is key to point out that the arachidonic acids that all fats eventually become are dependent of their own built in enzymes. Arachidonic acid (AA) is NOT found in these commercially accepted oils and lards. AA is needed to break down the stearic acid (which we mentioned earlier is necessary for a normal metabolism) in our animal fats, but since it isn't there to do this in processed fats, we have a problem. This lack of AA is the link that leads to blocking the conversion of PG1 and 3's into good (life saving) hormones. Again, because animal fats have this component, they are safe. It is foods like creamy peanut butter, commercial snack foods and French fries you need to avoid.

Those foods contain fake fats, hydrogenated oils, and trans-fatty acids that are NOT acceptable by any means. Meat is alright. Get it now? Sure, you should limit your animal fat intake (by trimming your steak marbles, shedding the skin off your chicken, tossing out a few egg yolks, etc), but do not limit your animal protein sources. Protein assists PG1 and 3's in doing their jobs and converting into healthy hormones! I know, I know, I know, you love your peanut butter. So do I! In it's natural form, peanut butter is fine. But after it is processed, creamed, hydrogenated and then having had sugar added to it, it's now B-A-D. Here is why. Hydrogenated fats (lards) in addition to sugar, alcohol, smoking, stress, toxicity, low protein diets and many other factors all block the enzyme delta 6 desaturase.

This enzyme is essential in turning our good fats into PG1 and PG3 hormones. And what happens to a blocked fat? They get stored as cellulite (nasty adipose tissue). That's what makes your butt all dumpy and gross. Hydrogenated oils. And that's not all. In a relatively healthy individual, it takes 7 weeks for hydrogenated oils to exit the body. And since good fats only last 3 weeks inside of you, quitting the program in under 2 months is hardly enough time to be cleaned out enough. Try this program for the length of time I recommended earlier so that you can see I'm right.

That's also why it takes consistent daily supplementation to replace essential fats and why I say it's at least 21 to 49 days for all the positive changes to be realized by some folk on this program. You're toxic folks! Face it! So if you get a little bloated, experience a little exhaustion or have a headache or two, you know why. The toxins have entered your bloodstream on their way out of the body.

No matter what, do not take any drugs to alter this process. Aspirin, acetaminophen and other anti-inflammatory drugs (like ibuprofen) will pose further problems. These drugs are beneficial only for a short time because they block the negative workings of the PG2 group. However, they also interfere with the PG1 and PG3's. This is why you will burn fat for a little while using those "ECA" stacks but then almost over night, it all stops. What could you do to clear out toxins and hydrogenated oils from your body a little faster? Start incorporating olive oils into your diet. Cook with it and pour it on your green vegetables. Omega 9 fats are great for cleansing the liver. All of your other essential fats can be gathered by incorporating 2 egg yolks, a tablespoon or two of Lemmon's Oil, olive oil, real butter and 2 tablespoons of raw cream a day. That's about 30 to 40 grams of very HEALTHY fat. Fat that makes you lean and mean, not fat like a cat! I used to recommend a product that was fairly close to what we need but I use my own blend of oils these days. I do not trust anyone else to make them anymore.

I am truly tired of the light colored blends which claim they are something they aren't. My oil is a unique blend of several different fatty acid sources. It meets the demands set forth in this chapter and is not only richer, but thicker, tastier and more nourishing than any other oil you know. It is also fresher by leaps and bounds too. That's right.

You can forget about using oil that is 6 to 12 month old ever again (and that's what they are despite the manufacturer's claim). You haven't lived until you have used an oil freshly pressed just 7 days before you receive it. This oil is Lemmon's Oil. Why did I make my own oil? Well, as each year passed that I was recommending another product, I asked myself why I hadn't done it long time ago. The quality of the blend seemed to dwindle, it tasted more and more stale and the delivery time became far too unpredictable each passing month.

The customer service and the people who ran the company were nothing but a bunch of clowns. Bitter? Yes. Those people raped me and they are raping the public. Tired of being at someone else's mercy, I had all I could take so I put together something BETTER than whatever you are currently using because I felt it HAD TO be done. I couldn't go another month without proper essential fatty acid nourishment and many women I have had as clients weren't tolerating it any longer either.

When we first met, she was severely depleted of her fats. And trust me, you only know what you are missing when you start using a good oil then stop taking it. So, what I did was contact the most reputable natural oil company in North America and explained my situation. Seems my complaints with the previous manufacturer were more than common knowledge in the industry. We moved forward and the result is Lemmon's Oil, which contains only Omega-flo unrefined certified organic oils including:

High Lignan Flax Seed, Sunflower Seed, Safflower Seed, Pumpkin Seed, Borage Seed, Sesame Seed, Almond, Wheat Germ several other wonderful ingredients. The wheat germ oil is used as a source of octacosanol (500 mg of wheat germ oil provides 1000 mcg of octacosanol) and rice bran oil for gamma oryzonol (which contains ferulic acid). Both of these oils have shown positive results in increasing glycogen storage and assisting in effective carbohydrate metabolism (with just 2 grams per 100 pounds of body weight a day).

My oil is high in natural antioxidants, FIBER, blood cleansing and emulsifying ingredients.

When I say it is THICKER, TASTIER, more nourishing and FRESHER than any other oil available, you really aren't going to fully appreciate it until you try some. It truly is the most complete source of essential fatty acids I know of anywhere. This product is the highest source of usable Omega 3 oils available because of the specific mixture and ratios. What we have here is a unique blend that falls into the most natural balance of nearly 50% Omega 3's, only 10% but all healthy saturated fat sources, and just above 20% of both omega 6's and 9's. The dark brown and greenish color of "Lemmon's Oil" displays its flora/vegetation origins.

A far cry from the pale colors the competition offers. If you use this oil and this oil alone, no other oil is necessary in the human diet... Because nothing else compares and you won't pay for expensive glass either. Lemmon's Oil is manufactured with an exclusive low temperature pressing (86 to 99 degrees F, 30 to 37 degrees C) and the processing and packaging (HDPE) is performed in complete exclusion of light, oxygen and reactive metals to maintain the life of the Omega Fatty Acid nutrients. There are no additives, no preservatives, no bleaching agents and no hexane extraction involved in its production. No trans fatty or hydrogenated fatty acids are found in Lemmon's Oil either.

Only certified organic seeds and completely unrefined oils that were not genetically modified are used in MY oil. We use Lemmon's Oil as a condiment on meats and vegetables after cooking them or on my salads and cottage cheese. Sometimes I even have a tablespoon by itself. The taste is a wonderful mix of buttery, nutty, and tangy flavors and it's really smooth going down! Adopt this oil as a regular part of your nutrition plan and you will never go astray again. Vitamins are like a good football team. You need a full team of vitamins on the field every time the ball is in play.

The ball is your life. Sometimes we keep other vitamins from the roster on the bench, watching those on the field, waiting their turn. Each member of your team knows what to do when the time comes and each player has a different job from the others. A good team doesn't bully it's own players nor feed off other members. Each works with its teammate's strengths without depleting itself because vitamins look out for each other. All nutrients are meant to work together this way, and none really stand alone, no matter how important you think they are.

If one vitamin is missing, or if one is in too high of a dosage, then somehow, some way, some where, it disrupts the team. This is what weakens your support structure. Minerals are different from vitamins because they are more like having fans in the stadium. Without fans, there really isn't any support for your team. In other words, there is no motivation for the vitamins to work their hardest without minerals. While some of the minerals are more visible and exciting than the others and may appear to be more important, kind of like cheerleaders, without even just one row of fans sitting in the stands, you can easily tell that something is missing. The support will not be there like it used to be, and it will show. Even if you do not know what it is for sure that is missing at first, something is definitely not right, and it could cost you the game. What pulls the team together, what pulls the best of all teams together, is coaches.

You and I both know that a team without direction gets nowhere. Well, fats are the coaches, trainers and administration that normally go uncredited for pulling the vitamin team together and gathering the fan support of the minerals for a winning effort.

The fans love them for what they do, the team needs them to digest and assimilate their orders correctly, so without having a good foundation of coaches, everything falls apart. You NEED fats. Especially essential fats.... And Lemmon's Oil provides ALL of them.... And if you are interested in trying Lemmon's Oil, if you haven't already, it comes in a 16 oz bottle that yields 32 servings of 120 calories each (these calories DO count in your overall caloric intakes but these fats DO NOT make you fat) and we will be glad to make some fresh for you.

When your muscles do not have enough glycogen which is made from carbohydrates, your endurance is shot, you get fatigued and not only will performance drop, your progress will not exist. How can you assure glycogen is spared? Having enough essential fatty acids available at all times. Follow this rule and in no time at all you will become a physical specimen to behold....

Why should you get your EFAs from Lemmon's and not Fish Oil? Although fish oil also contains EFAs, it actually has much less omega-3 EFA than Lemmon's oil primary ingredient Flax Seed Oil (let's not forget the other ingredients that cause the synergistic effect that elevates Lemmon's Oil above your flax seed oil standing alone). Also, fish oil is high in cholesterol (a sterol found exclusively in animals) and may contain detectable heavy metals and contaminants. See PerfectEFAOilBlend.com

One question I get a lot is: "Dear Don, I have been hearing flax seed oil is not good for you. Is this true?" Answer: Plain and simple, those rumors are spread by people who are selling fish oil because they know their product isn't as good so they stoop to media lies... Our source of flax is the purest in North America.

TAKING VITAMINS AND MINERALS

Exactly what role does your health really play in your lifestyle? Are you kidding? It is everything. But if you continue to look after your health for the next ten years as you have looked after it for the past ten years, what can you look forward to in the future? Is the quality of your life really important enough to you that you will make the necessary adjustments? Did you know that in many cases the reasons you cannot meet your goals, burn fat or build muscle nor slow down the aging process due to what's missing from the supplements you take? With the change from glucose as an energy source to using more free fatty acids and stored fat, toxins that were once stored in those fats are now ending up in your bloodstream. Just know, toxins WILL make you feel tired, sick, cranky, hungry, and etc. It's not the food, it's the junk left behind.

You need 'ANTIOXIDANTS' to remove these toxins (and other free radicals and waste products that are in there). No, you won't need a prescription to get them. Antioxidants are nothing more than vitamins and minerals that protect the body from free-radical damage. These toxins are partly to blame for wrinkles, cancer, pain and cramping that occur once cellular damage begins. An optimal antioxidant should be found to contain upwards of 200 I.U. of vitamin E (DE, not DLE. DL signifies synthetic, meaning not natural), 1000 or more mg of vitamin C and bioflavonoids, at least 7500 I.U. of beta carotene, 200 micrograms of selenium, and 15 to 30 mg of zinc. Wait a minute!

The Don Lemmon Multi-Nutrient contains exactly this already! How convenient! Other antioxidants and free radical scavengers like herbs are useful too. We include grape seed extract in ours for this reason but you can never be too careful that some huckster isn't trying to convince you gravel is an antioxidant these days too. Someone is bound to do this sooner or later. I remember when the amount of grape seed extract we use in our formula was $40 a bottle.

If it were worth $40 a bottle for exactly what we use, how could we afford to put 100 other nutrients in there for almost half the price? Because anything over priced is NEVER worth getting. It may benefit you, but there is no need to pay that much for it. Have you been taking other supplements because your joints hurt? I'm not so sure you should be wasting your money on overpriced snake oils, which supposedly prevent cancer as they heal joints. Fishes don't get cancer nor do they get hit by busses. From what I have learned on this subject, it's the plankton that fish eat which protects them from cancer, not their cartilage that most everything on earth is born with.

What plankton does is assist minerals into the cells of your tendons. Where are you going to get a ton of plankton on a daily basis anyhow? I certainly believe that other species' cartilage may relieve pain by strengthening your joints because eating chicken cartilage (yes, that's true) does. But cure CANCER? Based upon what? The fact the fish doesn't get cancer? Puh-lease. I would simply double my mineral intake, eat more chicken legs (skinless and not fried or breaded), start having more dark green veggies if not seaweed (which we buy as sushi paper wrap to roll rice with it or we get the weed itself and make soup). If that fails, I would begin taking an extra 500% of the RDA in B-6 and begin supplementing with some RUTIN until the pain subsides.

Rutin is a bioflavoniod from the pulp of citrus fruits that has displayed a role in healing tendons and ligaments in the old and young alike. It is also great for carpal tunnel syndrome. Wait a minute! The Don Lemmon Multi-Nutrient already has 1000% of the RDA in B-6 and contains a great source of rutin!

Who says I haven't covered the bases? All other remedies may fall by the wayside if we keep going at this rate! Even if you do find a product that works in curing disease, taking an antidote after taking a poison only works temporarily in delaying your demise.

Please address the other factors in your lifestyle which you know you should change because supplements do not remove the bad habits which caused the ailment. Getting back to nature, getting back to the basics, ALWAYS works, so let's do that. The other issue I have with supplements are diuretics and water pills. None of them do what the ads claim. While fat is less than 15% water and over 70% fat, and muscles are over 70% water and contain only 6% fat, guess where you'll lose weight from if you use diuretics or water pills?

From wherever the predominance of your water is stored, that's where! Muscle! If you are over 50, growth hormone therapy may help. In very low therapeutic dosages, HGH can help anyone, but in higher dosages, if you are below 40 especially, you are only looking for trouble. You won't see the negative side effects right away, just like with other drugs, that is if the HGH is synthetic, but in 20 years you will. If the form you use requires a needle to inject, look out! You know how a liver donor has to match blood types? Or a kidney needs to come from a relative?

What makes you think that any old source of HGH from some dead person you do not even know, or a cow for that matter, will be tolerated by your body any differently than that? I know most of you will think you need more "stuff" than I recommend, or that I am only trying to sell my own products, but really, you do not need much else. Some other supplements serve a purpose, but usually they are used for limited time and they only work if the product is of the same quality used in clinical studies. More often than not, you can't get that quality. Go buy something you think is supposed to work. You'll see. Especially once your diet becomes secure. That's because if you eat right, nothing except what I have told you about is necessary. Isn't eating right and taking vitamins good enough then? Sure, eating right does wonders, but food isn't what it used to be. That's why we must adhere to so many rules in order to succeed on food alone.

Our soils are depleted year after year from farming, pesticides and hormones leach ever more from what we eat and in most cases, the food is aged by time we have even the freshest of sources ready to consume. Sometimes, it's got at the most a 50th of what food had 50 years ago. No kidding. And what do you think happens when you cook your food? It gets fresher?

Our crops have 98% less of some of the same nutrients in them today as the crops grown in our same U.S. soils using the same testing techniques in 1948. It only takes 10 years of intensive farming to exhaust the minerals in any tract of land. Some of the major farms haven't rested their fields in over 50 years. Besides all that, even the best of vitamins only cover 20% of the necessities your body requires believe it or not. And while taking any old vitamin may help a little if you're really deficient, it is still not going to help you enough unless you also get ALL of your minerals and make sure the nutrients are in proper ratios to one another.

These are the keys along with eating right and getting essential fatty acids that assist your nutrients. Minerals and dosages are what make the difference between any old vitamin and a good product. Vitamins are essential organic compounds. And various amounts of each vitamin participate in the functions of the entire human body. This includes growth, fat loss, mental acuity, disease prevention and energy production. Some vitamins are fat-soluble (meaning they require fat to process) like A, D, E and K. Other vitamins are water-soluble vitamins like the various B-Complexes, C and such (meaning if you are dehydrated, they do not function properly). Vitamins generally cannot be synthesized by the body unless you deplete yourself of other nutrients to do so. The only time the body makes it's own is when you have crossed that 'danger' zone and are heading into severe malnourishment. The thing is, they cannot be made in adequate amounts under these conditions and this is why they absolutely MUST be supplied by your eating and supplementation habits.

These nutrients became publicly known around 1912 when Vitamin A was first isolated. The others were found one by one up until 1948 or so when B12 was discovered. The term 'vitamin' stems from a reference to the fact these nutrients are 'vital' because the body is fallible without them. Vitamins come mostly from plants and grains except for vitamins B, C and D, which are present in the muscle tissue of animals that consume foods containing them. Considering that only about one-quarter of the people reading this will ever eat correctly each and every day, and since vitamin critics don't adequately recognize deficiencies of the average diet, or what it takes to regain what we have lost, you had better take this seriously.

Each vitamin has specific work to perform inside of you and a deficiency of one vitamin cannot be remedied by consuming more of another. This is another reason why a variety of foods should be consumed on a daily basis. You need a little of everything, not too much or too little of anything. Natural vitamins are those occurring in food from animal or plant sources. Synthetic vitamins are usually identical to natural vitamins and if taken with food, the body will recognize them as part of the food. However, a few synthetic vitamins do differ from their natural forms.

Synthetic Vitamin E, called dl-alpha-tocopherol, is a mixture of both left and right handed molecules so to speak, while the natural E alpha-tocopherol is a single molecule form called d-tocopherol. The synthetic product is adjusted so that it provides the same biological activity as the natural form. They do this because it's common knowledge people do not eat as good as they should. They think simply popping pills is all they have to do. "But Doctor, I take a multi-vitamin daily." Really? Does it contain minerals? ALL minerals? Minerals are completely different inorganic (non-carbon containing) nutrients that also cannot be formed in the body and must be obtained from the diet.

Minerals are either positively charged (cations) or negatively charged (anions). Cations are derived from metal elements such as calcium, cobalt, chromium, copper, iron, magnesium, manganese, molybdenum, potassium, selenium, sodium and zinc. Anions are derived from non-metallic elements such as iodine, sulfur, phosphorus, chlorine, and fluoride (to name a few). Combining anions and cations together synergistically creates mineral salts such as sodium chloride, calcium phosphate and sodium iodide.

And as much as minerals work, play or belong together, vitamins and minerals are even more dependent of one another than minerals are of each other. You know how some football players are bigger than others? A lineman may be 300 pounds but a quarterback is probably 225? Or a receiver is 185 pounds and a running back might weight 200 pounds? All nutrients follow the same suit. Each 'player' so to speak has a specific daily task that requires a certain amount of support at all times. If a lineman weighed only 200 pounds he would probably get eaten up by the opposing team pretty quick and would be unable to do his job. If a quarterback weighed 185 pounds he would get crushed. If a receiver weighed 300 pounds he would be too large to get his work done.

This is why without a properly formulated multi-nutrient that contains all the vitamins and all the minerals in ratios or weights that allow them to work efficiently, you'll survive, but you won't feel, look or live up to your potential. I used to take a multiple vitamin that contained exactly 100% of the RDA dosages of all the major vitamins. I thought my body needed a little more so I took it twice a day. Well, in time, this proved not to be enough. Why? One, no minerals, and two, like I said, because we require more or less of certain nutrients. Sure, you may think if you take more than the RDA recommends, the vitamins or minerals will become toxic inside of you but when a person's body is trying to heal, up to 10 times the RDA may be required for a number of different nutrients.

The other reason that I stopped using my old vites was that some nutrients can't be taken in 100% of the RDA and expected to benefit you. Sometimes that is way too much. Vitamins are definitely something that should be taken with meals at least twice a day. There are around 20 essential vitamins you need so like I said, simply popping a Vitamin C once in a while or taking any old multi-vitamin or 'once-a-day' caplet is not going to cut it.

I have gone to great lengths in discussing nutrition in this book so far. What I have said may surprise many in the fitness industry as well as the folks who aren't in the industry. And while there are still those of you who refuse to eat right no matter what I say and insist that if you take supplements you read about in an article somewhere that you will still somehow get somewhere, you're entirely incorrect. First of all, you must eat right. Eating bad isn't remedied by popping pills, even if it is my pills. You have to eat right or the body cannot assimilate anything you take. In fact, only once you get your diet together, then and only then should you add supplements.

Next, tell me something. Is the multi-vitamin you are using now a caplet? I suggest that you begin CHEWING your pills if they are caplets. The coating of most pills is typically too hard to digest and your gut cannot break them down. As undesirable as that may seem to chew these things, you might as well get used to it. You will appreciate the fact that the pill doesn't come right back out your tail end anymore either. Oh, sorry. You didn't know that most caplets end up coming through you unused? That's right. Like I said, the coating is too tough for the enzymes in your belly to break apart.

This is why the product I use comes in a soft gel capsule. My product, which I have personally created, is an all natural, patented, and exclusive blend manufactured for me under the strictest of supervision. It was designed using my own research and is based upon clientele feedback and blood tests.

The nutrients are in ratios I feel not only enhance the bio-availability of all the other nutrients but increase the uptake of the foods we eat. That's what makes my particular product invaluable! There is literally nothing like it anywhere. What we have available to us now is a blend of pure science, technology, and essential metabolic function that not only meets, but exceeds my expectations to a point that I have changed my opinion on what I think of the competition. There is no competition.

You can literally feel the results taking this product the first day. When was the last time you could say that? The only way I can explain it is that you will feel a sort of mental clarity when you first take them. It's an incredible sensation. You will actually feel rejuvenated without feeling like you have drank a pot of coffee. No jitters cause there's no stimulants. Just proper nutrition. How is that possible? There are at least 90 of the nearly 100 naturally occurring and essential elements known to man in my product. That's 90% of your nutrition folks. All that's missing are your fats but you get those from Lemmon's Oil. A daily serving of the Official Don Lemmon Multi-Nutrient Formula (these capsules, not horse pills or caplets) provides:

Vitamin A (Beta Carotein Seaweed/Palmitate), 7500 IU: This nutrient is involved in vision, smell, hearing, taste, reproduction, adrenal and thyroid glands, metabolic rate, energy, body temperature, skin, and infections in the throat. It also affects lungs, digestive tract, and wound healing. Yes, it is an Anti-Oxidant (fights the free radicals and toxins which scavenge our cells).

Vitamin C (Calcium Ascorbate), 500 mg: Those deficient in this nutrient bruise easily and their blood vessels are so weak that their gums bleed when brushing them even lightly. Vitamin C is an antioxidant too that stimulates the adrenal glands to manufacture cortisone, which is involved in healing and helps to combat stress.

It supports immunity by stimulating the production of white blood cells and fights viral and bacterial infections. Vitamin C normalizes blood pressure, lowers cholesterol, thins the blood, and protects you from atherosclerosis and other forms of heart disease.

Vitamin B1 (Thiamine Mononitrate), 20 mg: B complex vitamins smell because they contain sulfur and nitrogen. If you take oral contraceptives, you are deficient in B1. It is also required for carbohydrate metabolism, along with B2, B3 and B5. B1's responsible for nerve, heart, muscle and digestive tissue health.

Vitamin B2 (Riboflavin), 7 mg: Exercise, pharmaceuticals and consistent sinus problems are signs we require more B2. It is also responsible for converting protein into amino acids. Vitamin G was the original name for riboflavin (B2).

Vitamin B3 (Niacinamide), 50 mg: This is the best form of niacin to take because it doesn't make your face red and flushed. B3 metabolizes bad triglycerides and lowers the risk of cancer.

NOTE: Vitamin B-4 (Adenine) is currently not considered an essential nutrient because it is readily available in grains and cereals. This nutrient must be present in the diet in order for the body to produce adenosine triphosphate (ATP).
Vitamin B5 (d-Calcium Pantothenate), 100 mg: Essential for the synthesis of steroid hormones naturally found in the body including adrenal hormones. In highly stressed situations, more B5 is better than 'just' enough especially if you suffer from allergies. People suffering from rheumatoid arthritis have decreased levels of B5.

Vitamin B6 (Pyrodoxine HLC) 20 mg: B-6 controls temper tantrums, mood swings, PMS, carpal tunnel syndrome and a number of mental disorders, including clinical depression and schizophrenia.

B6 depletion has also been connected to immune deficiency, kidney disease, asthma, sickle cell anemia and diabetes.

Biotin 250 mcg: Also known as Vitamin B7 or Vitamin H but it is actually just biotin. However, biotin is essential for metabolizing and controlling protein, fats, carbs, blood sugar, amino, lactic and pyruvic acids. It also aids in the prevention of hair loss so it is good to take a little more. Because it is water-soluble, any excess is excreted through the urine.

Folate (Folic Acid), 400 mcg: Folate is B8 which is Folic Acid B9 which kind of is Folacin or B11 that is yet another form of folic acid too. This nutrient is essential for red blood cell division and immunity.

Alcoholics, pregnant women, people who eat fast foods and the elderly all benefit from this vitamin.

Vitamin B10 aka PABA (Para Amino Benzoic Acid), 30 mg: This nutrient is for stress and relaxes you without putting you to sleep. PABA aids healthy bacteria, the formation of red blood cells, protects against the sun, and returns prematurely gray hair to its natural color. It is depleted during times of constipation.

Vitamin B12 (Cyanacobalamin), 400 mcg: B-12 is important in healing ligament and disc problems, energy, surgical recovery, anemia, cancer, insomnia, vary forms of depression and stress. But B12 also requires iodine and manganese to process. Laxatives, alcohol, aspirin, antibiotics, diuretics, antacids, caffeine, cooking and being not eating meat all cause us to be malnourished of B12.

They say B12 in the form of methylcobalamin is more absorbable but I am not convinced of this.

NOTE: Vitamin B13 (Orotic acid) is primarily used for the metabolization of folic acid and vitamin B12.

It is found in root vegetables and is good for multiple sclerosis and liver-related complications, which leads to premature aging. However, the FDA does not consider it vital for human beings and it is banned from dietary supplements as it is suspected of being carcinogenic.

Vitamin B15 (Pangamic Acid) is also not included as the body only needs it if you are a serious alcoholic or someone with degenerative liver problems that only your physician can diagnose. They may refer to it as the 'hangover' helper.

Vitamin B16 (Amygdalin) is also sometimes known as laetrile or B17 is a nutritional compound of two sugar molecules, (benzaldehyde and cyanide). It is used in an unaccepted form of cancer treatment. This B vitamin is the only one that is not found in brewer's yeast. Despite being found abundantly in fruits and green veggies, due to divided medical opinions, it is not included in this particular supplement.

Choline (Bitartrate), 450 mg: This partner in the B-Complex family works well with essential fatty acids. It improves short-term memory in normal, senile and people in the beginning stages of Alzheimer's Disease. Certain regions of the brain are easily depleted of acetylcholine especially. Diet doesn't boost the level of choline in the brain at all, and without it, most other nutrients cannot reach the brain either.

Inositol, 200 mg: Another B-Complex family member, inositol promotes alpha adrenergic activity which benefits the heart's coronary vessels, clearing cholesterol and burning body fat.

Look, you may feel nothing is missing from 'your' diet and supplements aren't 'essential' but do the math. B-Complexes are quite important. People are recommended to take B-complex vitamins for their allergies, anxiety, acne, adrenal support, arthritis, bursitis, bowel disorders, bruising, cramps, cardio ailments, depression, dermatitis, diabetes, and even epilepsy.

Do B12 'shots' ring a bell? You're depleted.

Vitamin D (Cholecalciferol), 300 IU: Fungus on the feet? Stinky bowel? You're deficient. Vitamin D detoxifies, prevents PMS and breaks down carbohydrates. Many elderly people are deficient in this vitamin, probably due to a lack of sunlight, but more likely due to dietary depletion. Crohn's disease, epilepsy, high blood pressure, kidney disease, liver disease, osteoporosis, and skin ailments are prevalent in vegetarians and those who do not get their fair share of the Big D.

Vitamin E (tocopherol blend), 200 IU: Vitamin E delays many effects of aging, prevents fibrocystic breast disease, edema (fluid retention), is essential in blood clots, scar tissue, burns, headaches, and should always be taken with proper amounts of selenium and Vitamin C. Without enough Vitamin E you can forget about Vitamin A doing it's thing.

NOTE: Vitamin F is a pet term for essential fatty acids like those in Lemmon's Oil. Also note, Vitamins B18 through B-gazillion and Vitamins I, J, L, etc aren't anything to concern ourselves with so I won't be covering them here...

Vitamin K (Phytonadione), 50 mcg: Antibiotics deplete the body of vitamin K. Ever taken an anti-biotic? Did you know it could take YEARS to replace what those drugs deplete? Vitamin K is found in dark green vegetables.

Bioflavinoids (Rutin, Quercitin), 500 mg: While technically not vitamins, 50 different bioflavinoids are found in the pulp of citrus fruits, in pine bark and even grape seeds. They act as antioxidants and are natural tendon and ligament healers that are also dandy anti-inflammatory agents.

Vitamin "P" as they were first known are not essential but if you have aches and pains in your joints, you're going to love us for including them.

Boron (Chelate),10 mg: This mineral is required for the maintenance of bone and normalizing blood levels of estrogen and testosterone. In fact, within a week ladies, you will lose less than half the calcium, a third less magnesium and twenty five percent less phosphorus through your urine than you are used to just by taking this supplement.

Calcium (Citrate/ Chelate), 500 mg: If you are deficient, the thyroid gland fails as the body begins absorbing it from the intestines and bones. You don't want that. And you know those canker sores that develop on the inside of your mouth? They are related to a calcium deficiency too. Canker sores are a form of the herpes virus. Once you have it, you have it forever but if you keep your calcium levels up...

The virus won't manifest canker sores. And keep in mind, calcium deposits are not caused from having too much calcium in the diet but from a lack of what is needed to process it... That's other minerals and B-complex vitamins!

Chloride (Potassium Chloride), 340 mg: Potassium chloride helps acidify tissues in people when their joints and bursae sacs ache (bursitis). It activates numerous enzymes and is the basic raw material for our stomachs to make stomach acid (HCl) for protein digestion (pepsin - a protease enzyme).

Chromium (Polynicotinate/Chloride), 300 mcg: This does what they say it does. It helps keep blood sugar levels steady so you can fight off cravings for sugar and carbohydrates while burning fat.

Chromium is a mineral that dieters seem to get a little obsessed over but you do not need more chromium in your diet as much as you need all the other minerals. If you insist on taking chromium, use 300 mcg of chromium poly-NICOTINATE (GTF) not picolinate for every 100 pounds of lean mass you carry.

Copper (Gluconate), 2 mg: Many times PMS, candida albicans, and even anemia disappears once a woman overcomes her copper deficiencies. Men, this nutrient is wonderful for the prostate.

Iodine (Kelp/Potassium Iodine), 150 mcg: Iodine is required if like certain people, you have recurrent sinus infections. This stems from an over active thyroid using up your iodine. Iodine will also adjust vaginal discharge.

Iron (Chelate), 4 mg: Symptoms of iron deficiency include listlessness, fatigue, heart palpitations, reduced cognition, memory deficits, sore tongue, angular stomatitis, dysphagia, and hypochromic microcytic anemia. Do you know anyone who chews ice? It is a disorder more commonly known as pagophagia. It stems from iron deficiency anemia. They probably have other cravings for red meats and even some non-food items. Do you or they also chew ink pens and fingernails? You need minerals. That's all. It goes away within the first few days of supplementation. If you are told that iron causes heart attacks, your source is misinformed. The iron we chose to use helps build red blood cells to carry oxygen throughout your body to shuttle the other nutrients to cells for energy and recuperation.

Magnesium (Citrate/Chelate), 450 mg: This nutrient is essential for calcium and potassium assimilation, contributes to proper nerve and muscle impulses and assists in the correction of nervousness, muscle weakness, heart palpitations, light headiness, diarrhea, most hormonal issues.

Fluoride from tap water and toothpaste, refined sugar and corn syrup and artificial sweeteners will deplete you of magnesium in a heartbeat. Magnesium carbonate, chloride and oxide are inorganic forms and are less absorbable than the chelated citrate we use.

Manganese (Gluconate), 10 mg: No, this isn't magnesium listed twice. This nutrient helps the thyroid gland produce hormones, speeds the metabolism function and without it Vitamin C and the B-complexes cannot do their jobs.

Molybdenum (Chelate), 75 mcg: It has been claimed that molybdenum influences the susceptibility to esophageal cancer. Studies suggest that cancer patients are deficient in molybdenum.

Phosphorous (di Calcium Phosphate), 100 mg: A phosphorus deficiency leads to not only osteoarthritis, but kidney stones, urinary tract and tartar on your teeth.

Selenium (l-Selenomethionine), 200 mcg: Also very helpful in preventing herpes outbreaks, preventing cellular mutation, cancers and if you are in treatment for AIDS, try taking 2,000 mcg of selenium daily

Vanadium (Vanadyl Sulfate), 150 mcg: Vanadium improves insulin action, inhibits formation of cholesterol in blood vessels and in the nervous system and improves the mineralization of bones and teeth.

Vanadyl Sulfate is a tool used by athletes to store extra glycogen, or sugar, inside the muscle for a more pumped look which could also contribute to greater strength (the extra glycogen, not the pump). Problem is, that doesn't work. The key word is EXTRA.

Vanadyl doesn't help one bit with what the body can already handle on its own in storing carbs really. If you're already full of intra-muscular carbohydrates, then and only then will the body accept any assistance. But if you're full, you're FULL. You can get all the Vanadyl you need from my multi-nutrient and 100 other nutrients at a greatly reduced price than buying Vanadyl alone anytime.

Zinc (Gluconate/Sulfate), 30 mg: Zinc helps with sexual function, mood stability, immunity and prevents body odor.

Grape Seed Extract (95% standardized OPC), 25 mg: OPC's are very powerful bioflavonoids that are assimilated into our body tissues and strengthen the blood within hours!

Essential Amino Acid Blend, 100 mg: Amino Acids are the "building blocks" of the human body. Besides doing all of the above, plus building cells, repairing tissue, forming antibodies, combating bacteria, viruses, being a part of the enzyme and hormonal systems, building RNA and DNA, carrying oxygen throughout the body filled with vitamins and minerals, what don't they do? There are eight amino acids considered essential because they cannot be manufactured by the body and for the sake of better nutrition, here they are. It's not a lot, but it's plenty to do what we need them to. Assist the other nutrients.

Dimethylglycime (DMG), 25 mg: This is another amino acid that specifically stimulates T-cell production, thus its job is to maintain the immune system.

Polyfloramin, 100 mcg: What the heck is this? It is the trademarked name given to the phytogenic extracts used exclusively in T. J. Clark Mineral products. It is basically all that is good taken from their exclusive blend of plant source trace minerals.

How do you like that? That's a lot of stuff isn't it? Well, it's all of your major vitamins, minerals, plus more B-Complex 'stress' vitamins Anti-Oxidants and trace minerals than any other product like this. Did you like that I have also included essential amino acids? There is just enough in there to make sure all the other nutrients have 'back up' to do their jobs!

I also used to take extra trace minerals on top of my regular vitamin and mineral supplementation, but not any more. Can you believe on top of it all, this particular formula contains a full day's serving of colloidal minerals? Like I said, no corners cut, nothing left out, all bases are covered! That's over 120 total nutrients using this system! Aren't you excited? When we got our first batch I felt like dancing, hitting the gym, going for a run, something... And I truly believe that the key to it all was the extra trace (colloidal) minerals we threw in. Why colloidal minerals though? What makes them so special? We know the major minerals build bone, muscle tissue, and support the nervous system.

Colloidal minerals promote the utilization of major minerals like calcium (boron) in saving your bones, the breakdown of sugar and carbohydrates (chromium), the building of red blood cells (cobalt), stronger teeth (with natural fluoride), enhancing thyroid function (iodine), fighting cancer (manganese), protein synthesis (molybdenum), fighting free radicals (selenium) and they even have antibiotic capabilities which help heal wounds by producing white blood cells (zinc). And this is just a short list.

The following colloidal minerals are found in Don Lemmon's Multi Nutrient Formula: Antimony, Arsenic, Aluminum, Barium, Beryllium, Bismuth, Boron, Bromine, Cadmium, Carbon, Cerium, Cesium, Chromium, Cobalt, Dysprosium, Erbium, Europium, Fluorine, Gadolinium, Gallium, Germanium, Gold, Hafnium, Holmium, Hydrogen, Iridium, Iron, Lanthanum, Lithium, Lutetium, Neodymium, Nickel, Niobium, Osmium, Oxygen, Palladium, Platinum, Praseodymium, Rhenium, Rhodium, Rubidium, Ruthenium, Samarium, Scandium, Silicon, Silver, Strontium, Tantalum, Tellurium, Terbium, Thallium, Thorium, Tin, Titanium, Tungsten, Vanadium, Ytterbium, Yttrium, and Zirconium.

Still don't think vitamins and minerals go together? Look at a bottle of Anti-Oxidants sometime.

You will not only notice that these products consist of both vitamins and minerals but my product supplies more nutrients than anyone else's does. The fact remains, a proper supplement is made up of both vitamins AND minerals, not just one or the other.

And if I can squeeze 120 nutrients in every single capsule, who do those other companies think they are fooling with their formulations? They only hold back what they offer you in their products so they can force you to feel the need to buy more than one product! It's simple marketing! They are cutting you short on purpose! Notice anything else in Don Lemmon's Multi-Nutrient that you have been buying separately and paying an arm and a leg for up until now? Well, don't do it anymore! People that are taking lithium for depression can find it here for pennies! Chromium? It's in there! Colloidal silver? We got it! Vanadium for carbohydrate metabolism? That is in there too! Amazing isn't it? No need to buy 50 different products every month. Take just this one multi-nutrient combined with Lemmon's Oil and you're all set.

Still think minerals are unnecessary? Got tartar on your teeth? That's a bonafide phosphorus deficiency. Take this product for a month and see if it helps or not. It will. And if you are a sweater, you are acidic. So not only do you need more minerals because you perspire more than most, but you need more minerals to stop the sweating, or at least control it. It's just another common mineral deficiency. No, Gatorade doesn't even come close to lending a hand (I have to laugh at that one)!

Even Dr Linus Pauling, the 2 time Nobel Prize winner in medicine and the King of the Vitamin C movement said "Every sickness, every disease, every ailment known to man can be traced to a mineral deficiency." Top that. Do you suffer from neuralgias, psychoses, eczema, poor sleep, lupus, herpes, hot flashes, obesity or any of the above?

Maybe you don't now, but later in life as you begin to age due to malnourishment you might. ALL these disorders are commonly associated with stress but it's really due to poor metabolism of B vitamins, not the actual lack of B-vitamins. It's a lack of the minerals needed to use the complexes. You bet, in fact, niacin and thiamin are totally useless without both minerals AND essential fatty acids in your system. So again, don't forget your Lemmon's Oil! Go team! Vitamins, minerals, trace nutrients, anti-oxidants, b-complexes, plus amino and essential fatty acids are the things that combine with your foodstuffs to create and maintain all your enzymes, cells, hormones, tissues, metabolic needs and even slows down aging. There isn't a function you can name that isn't protein, fat, vitamin or mineral dependant.

Many of the companies you recognize that sell vitamins and minerals dilute theirs with water, juices, sugars and other synthetic ingredients. This weakens your product. You can be certain that this particular product is free from artificial flavors, sweeteners, colors, corn, gluten, yeast, wheat, dairy, soy, preservatives or pesticides. This program is the Rolls Royce of nutrition AND health and you need your supplementation to complete it. You do DESERVE a Rolls Royce don't you?

If you are ready to try a full month supply of this Balanced Multi-Nutrient (180 capsules), simply drop me an email or visit BalancedMultiNutrient.com today! This product, originally called the Perfect Vitamin, along with Lemmon's Oil AKA the Perfect EFA Oil blend have been the nutritional foundation of this system since 2001. The oil alone is normally $20 and the multi $30. But through this book, both are being made available to you for just $39.95 a month! Contact us today to place your order!

Carbohydrates, proteins, and fats. Vitamin, minerals, and essential fatty acids. Getting sleep, exercise and making sure what goes in one end comes out the other. You have learned plenty so far. Let's keep reading....

AMINO ACIDS AND GLANDULAR THERAPY

I remember my first bottle of amino acids like it was yesterday. I bought them for $20 from a guy named Robb Lee in Newton Falls, Ohio where I grew up. He now owns a great restaurant there, but that is beside the point. These amino acids (protein pills) were made by a company that no longer produces the same goods, and smelled of pure ammonia. They say that is the highest of quality you will find anywhere. I thought I was taking something practically illegal and assumed it was going to make me a muscled bodybuilder overnight just by taking those stinky horse pills. Nothing happened though. I took the entire bottle in a month, 12 or 16 of them a day I think, and yet NOTHING HAPPENED.

I didn't realize I was supposed to start lifting weights to build the muscle. I hadn't a clue. That's the same attitude most people have. Pop a pill, the world becomes a better place. Supplements are supposed to assist you by being an 'extra' boost to your current plan. If the plan is not complete, it can only boost you so much. True for anything you try. If you take a fat burner that boosts your metabolism by 10%, it isn't going to show results if everything else you do continues to reduce the metabolism by 30% now is it? The aminos I first took only served to feed my malnourished body instead of helping it grow muscles. They couldn't possibly help to build even a little muscle.

I wasn't eating enough nor lifting weight to substantiate my body to grow. Six months later, after I was weight training regularly, the next products I tried were mega packs from the local health store. They had a deal where you bought two bags or bottles and they gave you another one free. These at least made a difference because they were my first source of real nutrition (I didn't eat very well). I was taking like 8 packs a day, 10 capsules of amino acids before, during and after my training too. I wasn't sure what worked, the training or the pills.

After a while, I noticed something stimulated my metabolism enough that I began eating more food and more often. Up to the point of eating more, I was getting muscular but wasn't putting on much weight. The next summer, I tried my first protein powder. I replaced fast food with protein powder. Again, I didn't get anywhere all week using it. In fact, I lost muscle that week.

Everyone in this industry wants to sell you treated powdered milk, fake sugars that cause disease, hydrogenated oils that interfere with healing and hormones, synthetic vitamins the body doesn't recognize, filtered and flavored minerals that are useless and pro hormones that the pros wouldn't even bother with. Everyone claims they sell only the best and they wouldn't tell a lie. Well, that's the smoke they are blowing up your skirt. As Willie Wonka once said "We are the dreamers of dreams." This is precisely what they depend upon. It wasn't until I had been training for several years that I stumbled across something that worked. I have just re-created the wheel folks...

I reinvented the SUPER STEROL COMPLEX...

When I decided to put together this product I was certain I took into consideration popular ingredients like beta sitosterol (sistosterol), adrenal and other glandular or botanical dietary supplements, how certain amino acids affected the liver, dessicated (desiccated) liver tablets as they are a mainstay or staple and then made sure that another key amino acid essential to liver function were used. After all, what's popular and what's scientifically sound go hand in hand, right? Not always...

If you have used Don Lemmon's KNOW HOW products before then you already know the level of professionalism, the quality of his ingredients and the beauty of his presentations. This product contains a 30 day supply of capsules and each ingredient in Don Lemmon's Glandular Complex has multiple benefits. Here are some very useful tid bits about all things it offers. Let's start with...

PHYTO-STEROLS: We discuss phyotosterols first so you can see how they compliment our other product, Lemmon's Oil and why we include them in this very special Glandular complex. Fats and proteins go together. Lemmon's Oil is a fat, so are sterols. The other ingredients we use are amino acids and glands defatted and dehydrated. These are the protein sources. So, to begin, phytosterols are plant fats similar in structure as the animal fat cholesterol, except they have an extra ethyl group on the side chain. All plants, including fruits, vegetables, grains, spices, seeds and nuts contain these sterol compounds or sterolins, with some of the most commonly found phytosterols being beta-sitosterol (BSS), stigmasterol, and campesterol. It is recognized that plant oils are a particularly rich source of phyto-sterols, however all sources are not the same while our selections are most effective in the treatment or prevention of high cholesterol, or hypercholesterolemia. What sets these compounds apart from many other phytonutrient products that boast similar health-promoting attributes is the success stories of people who have used these products.

The interest in the effects of phytosterols apparently started with Roelof Wilke Liebenburg from South Africa, who witnessed how one of his relatives with inoperable prostate cancer was supposedly cured by a neighbor using a traditional folk remedy. As a result, Mr. Liebenburg started researching the plant components that were used to treat his relative's cancer, and eventually a small study was done in Germany with patients suffering from a variety of prostate problems. Following the successful treatments of some cases with benign prostatic hypertrophy - or BPH (which is a non-cancerous enlargement of the prostate) by these plant extracts, a patented remedy of a special combination of sterols and sterolins was formulated in 1974. This product line was initially approved for BPH, however once it became available over-the-counter, it was touted as a most promising immune system cure.

With claims of alleviating asthma, diabetes, several types of cancers, herpes, rheumatoid arthritis, lupus, allergies, psoriasis, etc., etc.... It caught quite the buzz. Apparently, new research is also under way to confirm positive effects of phytosterols and sterolins on chronic fatigue syndrome, fibromyalgia, tuberculosis, sinusitis, HIV, Hepatitis C, and other infectious diseases, whereby beta-sitosterol in particular is said to modulate immune function, inflammation and pain levels through its effects on controlling the production of inflammatory cytokines. Research has also shown that phytosterols such as beta-sitosterol may help normalize the function of T-helper lymphocytes and natural killer cells following stressful events. Any positive effects of phyto-sterols on human cancers though are for legal reasons not able to be discussed at this time.

While test tube and other human studies showed impressive results of dietary phytosterols being able to lower serum cholesterol and slow the growth and spread of cancer cells, a number of human studies showed fairly good benefits in respect to alleviating the symptoms of benign prostatic hypertrophy (BPH). Of course, it was interesting to see how a diet maintaining clean sources of animal cholesterol fared - to which results appeared superior. I have followed the progress of a number of recent studies who had started using phytosterols for a variety of medical disorders that beta-sitosterol, stigmasterol, campesterol, or any number of other sterols or sterolins are supposed to be beneficial for.

At another point, I actually encouraged some clients to experiment with these products to help evaluate the effectiveness of phytosterols for their conditions. I also monitored my own chemistry while supplementing larger doses of sterols and sterolins myself in the hope of coming up with any specific positive or negative effects. Over the time I have been putting this product together there have been no negatives results regarding any number of medical conditions the products were used for.

Since everyday plant foods already contain adequate amounts of phytosterol compounds, extra supplementation would seem to benefit only those individuals who follow malnourishing diets that are low in calories, or where junk food rules their dietary life style. In such cases, either phytosterol supplementation or a better diet would be an option, although the thing to consider is that myself and my clients have all seen benefits on a highly nourishing diet. Here are the ones in my Glandular Complex.

Beta-Sitosterol - Over the past few years, concentrated extracts of this particular phytosterol have been tested for lowering cholesterol and lessening such discomforts of benign prostatic hyperplasia (BPH) as frequent and painful urination.

Behenic Acid - A constituent of most fats and fish oils. Large amounts are found in jamba, mustard seed, rapeseed oils, and cerebrosides. Also known as n-docosanoic acid, this is a fat that burns fat.

Beta-Ecdysone - Helps increase nitrogen retention and protein synthesis

Campesterol - Transporter expressed in the liver that regulates biliary sterol secretion. The observed inverse relation between hepatic clearance and intestinal absorption of cholesterol and campesterol supports the hypothesis that campesterol also supports intestinal sterol absorption.

Capsicum - Cannot be equaled by any known agent when a powerful and prolonged stimulant is needed, as in congestive chills, heart failure, and other conditions calling for quick action. The entire circulation is affected by this agent and there is no negative reaction.

Cytochrome C - Cytochrome c oxidase, the terminal enzyme in the respiratory chain, is located in the inner membrane of mitochondria and bacteria.

It catalyses the reduction of dioxygen to water and pumps an additional proton across the membrane for each proton consumed in the reaction. The resulting electro-chemical gradient is used elsewhere, for instance in the synthesis of ATP.

Dimethylglycine (DMG) - DMG helps the body to more efficiently utilize nutrients, and oxygen, at the cellular level. It can be used to ma-ntain good health, enhance performance and productivity as well as aid in the healing and restoration processes necessary to overcome a number of adverse health conditions. As a nutritional supplement, DMG can improve physical and mental performance by helping the body to adapt to various forms of stress, such as aging, poor oxygen availability, free radical damage, and a weakened immune system.

Deoxyribonucleic Acid (DNA) - A chemical substance found in chromosomes believed to be the substance that determines the manner in which healthy cells grow

Fucosterol - Show strong hypocholesterolemic activity. This ability to reduce 'bad' plasma cholesterol levels and to increase serum lipolytic (fat burning) activity may explain their use in the prevention of atherosclerosis. An antihypertensive activity of substances with sodium-binding properties, e.g. a polysaccharide is also observed with use.

Gamma Oryxanol - Gamma Oryzanol is a natural nutrient extract isolated from rice bran oil. Many individuals who are involved in weight-training as well as aerobic exercise programs are using Gamma Oryzanol as a natural steroid alternative to help develop lean muscle mass and improved definition and others use to rehab aging or injured tissues.

Inosine - Inosine belongs to a chemical family known as purine nucleotides. It penetrates cell walls of both cardiac and skeletal muscle and once inside promotes the manufacture of ATP, the substance in the body that allows muscles to contract.

Athletes wishing to exercise longer without experiencing muscle fatigue often use inosine. Inosine also promotes the production of a substance known as 2,3-DPG that is necessary for the transport of oxygen molecules from the red blood cells to the cell for energy. Japanese researchers have stated that inosine can be helpful for those with myocarditis, myocardiosclerosis, senile heart, cardiac arrhythmia and myocardial infarction.

Lignoceric Acid - A healthy saturated fatty acid that does not store as fat but is used directly in hormone regulation and energy production.

Methoxyisoflavone - It was determined that Methoxy Isoflavone is highly anabolic (increases protein synthesis) with no androgenic side effects. Meaning Methoxy Isoflavone throughout the studies has been shown to have no effect on the natural hormonal axis. This result along with the anabolic characteristic of the compound is fascinating. Methoxy Isoflavone has been identified to partially suppress the highly catabolic hormone, cortisone, while improving nitrogen retention by the body (additional proof of the anabolic effect.)

Myristic Acid - Impact of myristic acid versus palmitic acid on serum lipid and lipoprotein levels in healthy women and men has been touted as a remedy for those who do not process fat efficiently.

Octacosanol - Policosanol has been shown to normalize cholesterol as well or better than prescription cholesterol-lowering drugs, without side effects such as liver dysfunction and muscle atrophy. Efficacy and safety have been proven in numerous clinical trials, and it has been used by millions of people in other countries.

Policosanol - Lowers harmful LDL-cholesterol and raises protective HDL-cholesterol. HDL-cholesterol removes plaque from arterial walls.

Palmitic Acid - Recent studies have shown that the feeding of palmitic acid, a C16 fatty acid, results in an increase in the production of high density lipoprotein (HDL) cholesterol. In addition, the C16 fatty acid has been shown to be less hypercholesterolemic than the C12 to C14 fatty acids. Palm oil, also has the distinction of having more palmitic acid at the C-2 position of the glycerol component than any other common vegetable oil. It has been shown that infants thrive on fat formulas with a high palmitic content at the C-2 position.

Ribonucleic Acid (RNA) - Ribonucleic Acid is a complex protein that copies instructions for new protein production from the DNA genetic blueprints in the cell's nucleus, and carries those instructions to the cell's polyribosomes, where the new proteins are produced from materials already available and waiting.

Smilax Officinalis Extract - The method of this ingredient's action is less as a secernent than a sustainer of capillary circulation and its ultimate benefits are seen only after long use as a blood cleaner and nutrient carrier. If you want results, saturate the body for a prolonged period of time and do not stop.

Superoxide dismutase (SOD) - The main antioxidant in the eye lens. One of the body's two natural antioxidant enzymes. Zinc, copper, selenium and manganese are required for synthesis and are found in both this product and our Perfect Vitamin. Reduces high blood pressure and prevents cataracts. In animals of any species those with the highest level of SOD live the longest.

Stearic Acid - Research indicates that stearic acid is unique amongst the fat world. Unlike other saturated fats, stearic acid has a neutral effect on blood cholesterol similar to oleic acid, which is important when considering maintaining cardiovascular health. A proposed mechanism for the similarity between oleic acid and stearic acid is the rapid conversion of stearic acid to oleic acid by action of a delta-9 desaturase in the liver.

Stigmasterol - Assists in the conversion of linoleic acid to polyunsaturated fatty acids. This process is essential for the conversion of the Omega 6 fatty acids to prostaglandins and leukotrienes. Prostaglandins and leukotrienes are hormone like substances which are involved in immune support; they assist in the reduction of thrombo-embolic disorders by reducing platelet aggregation and they also assist in the reduction of inflammatory metabolites.

This product also contains a unique blend of DESICATED GLANDULARS. One of the basic concepts of glandular therapy is that the oral ingestion of glandular material of a certain and specific animal gland will strengthen the corresponding human gland. For instance, in case of infection of immune system deficiencies, thymus extracts and spleen extracts have been found to be quite useful. Glandular therapy has also been used extensively in the treatment of cancer and AIDS. On the other hand, if you have poor eyes or want to enhance already healthy eyes, you would ingest eye tissue of said animal. This of course would be disturbing to eat, and that is why we are providing the sources in desiccated forms for you with plenty of accessory nutrients to assist and multiply their benefits and use. The result is a broad general effect indicative of improved glandular function, fat loss, muscle building, health and digestion. Thus, glandular therapy increases the tone, function, and/or activity of the corresponding gland which benefits the entire human system. This principle is a mainstay of oriental therapy as are herbs (which is our other product, the Ultimate Herbal Formula).

Prior to the 1940s, glandular extracts were in wide use all over the world including the western world, and a considerable amount of research was in progress to support their use. With the development of antibiotics, and the advent of "modern" technological medicine, the research was concentrated on developing more and more antibiotics and other pharmaceutical drugs that was more profitable to the drug companies.

The research in glandular therapy came to a halt as a result. Just because the glandular approach was no longer being pursued in clinical research does not invalidate the usefulness of the approach or diminish the validity of its therapeutic value. It is still one of India's Ayurvedic Medicine.

In glandular therapy, purified extracts from the endocrine glands of animals are used to help restore a patient's overall metabolism. The extracts taken from animals are known clinically as protomorphogens. Protomorphogens are an important component of a complete nutritional program which as you can guess, is grossly neglected. They provide immediate as well as long term benefits. To date, typically glandular and organ extracts are indicated when a patient's endocrine system is underproducing or undersecreting a specific hormone or when an organ is weakened or diseased, such as is often the case with cancer patients. The treatment is generally recognized as effective. There are three principal nutritional benefits to glandular and organ extracts:

It is believed that glands and organs in animals and humans contain similar biochemical substances as their functions are very similar. This is especially true with the sheep from which most extracts are prepared. For example, sheep digestive system produces enzymes very similar to humans. Sheep tissue contains 2 enzymes found in only one other living organism-the human body. These enzymes are aldose reductase, an enzyme for sugar breakdown and steroid 17 -20 lyase, an enzyme for both producing steroidal hormones and for the subsequent detoxification of those hormones from the body. Thus, the effect of using the biochemical compounds extracted from animals is often one of "substituting" an exogenous (externally generated) source to make up for the endogenous (internally generated) deficiency. Glandular tissues are rich in many nutrients, including vitamins, minerals, amino acids, fatty acids, polypeptides, enzymes, and many other substances and this is why they work synergistically with all other products.

Glandular therapy can supply your missing essential nutritional needs in a highly efficient manner because keep in mind, for a tissue cell to repair or replace itself, it must have the raw materials necessary. Glandular therapy provides the raw materials to the failing organs, glands, and tissues so that they can start the process of regeneration. These products work because our glandular-based food supplements contain small polypeptide, protein-like substances which have specific messenger activity and which act on target tissues. Many of the hormones found in our own glandular tissues, even at low concentrations, still have potent tissue-specific activities if motivated. For example, a small polypeptide material present in one tissue can have selective effects in encouraging another tissue at a different site in the body to produce hormonal materials, which then may affect a final target tissue and change its physiological function.

Our Glandular Complex includes in sufficiently equal amounts: (from pure, clean and disease free lyophilized sources of Bovine, and Porcine glands)

Raw Adrenal Tissue Concentrate, Raw Aorta Tissue Concentrate, Raw Bone Marrow Tissue Concentrate, Raw Brain Tissue Concentrate, Raw Duodenum Tissue Concentrate, Raw Eye Tissue Concentrate, Raw Heart Tissue Concentrate, Raw Hypothalamus Tissue Concentrate, Raw Kidney Tissue Concentrate, Raw Liver Tissue Concentrate, Raw Lung Tissue Concentrate, Raw Lymph Tissue Concentrate, Raw Orchic Tissue Concentrate, Raw Pancreas Tissue Concentrate, Raw Parotid Tissue Concentrate, Raw Pituitary Tissue Concentrate, Raw Prostate Tissue Concentrate, Raw Spleen Tissue Concentrate, Raw Stomach Tissue Concentrate, Raw Thymus Tissue Concentrate, and Raw Thyroid Tissue Concentrate.

We round the product off with ESSENTIAL AMINO ACIDS.

These are the "building blocks" of the body. It is pure protein in raw form. Besides building cells and repairing tissue, amino acids form antibodies to combat invading bacteria & viruses, are part of the enzyme & hormonal system, build nucleoproteins (RNA & DNA), carry oxygen throughout the body and participate in muscle activity and muscular growth. When protein is broken down by digestion the result is 22 known amino acids. Eight are essential (meaning they cannot be manufactured by the body and must be taken orally) the rest are non-essential (meaning they can be manufactured by the body with proper nutrition but nonetheless have additional benefit when they are not required to be manufactured because that defeats the purpose).

CARNITINE (Non-Essential Amino Acid) - Carnitine and acetyl-l-carnitine play several important roles in the human body, particularly in energy metabolism. These nutrients shuttle acetyl groups and fatty acids into mitochondria for energy production. Without carnitine, fatty acids cannot easily enter into mitochondria. The acetyl group of acetyl-l-carnitine is used to form acetyl-CoA, the most important intermediary in the generation of energy from amino acids, fats, and carbohydrates. Therefore, acetyl-l-carnitine serves as an energy reservoir of acetyl groups and both acetyl-l-carnitine and carnitine help improve energy production.

GLUTAMINE (Non-Essential Amino Acid) - Glutamine helps the body maintain the correct acid-alkaline balance and is a necessary part of the synthesis of RNA and DNA. Glutamine also helps promote a healthy digestive tract. Unlike other amino acids that have a single nitrogen atom, glutamine contains two nitrogen atoms that enable it to transfer nitrogen and remove ammonia from body tissues. Glutamine readily passes the blood-brain barrier and, within the brain, is converted to glutamic acid, which the brain needs to function properly. It also increases the amount of GABA, which is needed to sustain proper brain function and mental activity.

ORNATHINE (Non-Essential Amino Acid) - Ornithine-a-Ketoglutarate, a powerful compound & precursor, has beneficial effect on hormones, the immune system, promotes healing in surgical and trauma cases and has anabolic properties.

TRYPTOPHAN (Essential Amino Acid) - A natural relaxant, helps alleviate insomnia by inducing normal sleep, reduces anxiety & depression, helps in the treatment of migraine headaches, helps the immune system; helps reduce the risk of artery & heart spasms; works with Lysine in reducing cholesterol levels.

LYSINE (Essential Amino Acid) - Insures the adequate absorption of calcium; helps form collagen (which makes up bone cartilage & connective tissues), aids in the production of antibodies, hormones & enzymes. Recent studies have shown that Lysine may be effective against herpes by improving the balance of nutrients that reduce viral growth. A deficiency may result in tiredness, inability to concentrate, irritability, bloodshot eyes, retarded growth, hair loss, anemia & reproductive problems.

METHIONINE (Essential Amino Acid) - Is a principle supplier of sulfur which prevents disorders of the hair, skin and nails, helps lower cholesterol levels by increasing the liver's production of lecithin, reduces liver fat and protects the kidneys, a natural chelating agent for heavy metals, regulates the formation of ammonia and creates ammonia-free urine which reduces bladder irritation, influences hair follicles and promotes hair growth.

PHENYLALAINE (Essential Amino Acid) - Used by the brain to produce norepinephrine, a chemical that transmits signals between nerve cells and the brain, keeps you awake & alert, reduces hunger pains, functions as an antidepressant and helps improve memory.

THREONINE (Essential Amino Acid) - Is an important constituent of collagen, Elastin, and enamel protein, helps prevents fat build-up in the liver; helps the digestive and intestinal tracts function more smoothly; assists metabolism and assimilation.

VALINE (Essential Amino Acid) - Promotes mental vigor, muscle coordination and calm emotions.

LEUCINE & ISOLEUCINE (Essential Amino Acid) - They provide ingredients for the manufacturing of other essential biochemical components in the body, some of which are utilized for the production of energy, stimulants to the upper brain and helping you to be more alert.

ARGININE (Non-Essential Amino Acid) - Studies have shown that is has improved immune responses to bacteria, viruses & tumor cells, promotes wound healing and regeneration of the liver, causes the release of growth hormones, and is considered crucial for optimal muscle growth and tissue repair.

TYROSINE (Non-Essential Amino Acid) - Transmits nerve impulses to the brain, helps overcome depression, improves memory, increases mental alertness, promotes the healthy functioning of the thyroid, adrenal and pituitary glands.

GLYCINE (Non-Essential Amino Acid) - Helps trigger the release of oxygen to the energy requiring cell-making process, important in the manufacturing of hormones responsible for a strong immune system.

SERINE (Non-Essential Amino Acid) - A storage source of glucose by the liver and muscles, helps strengthen the immune system by providing antibodies, synthesizes fatty acid sheath around nerve fibers.

GLUTAMIC ACID (Non-Essential Amino Acid) - Considered to be nature's "Brain food" by improving mental capacities, helps speed the healing of ulcers, gives a "lift" from fatigue, helps control alcoholism, schizophrenia and the craving for sugar.

ASPARTIC ACID (Non-Essential Amino Acid) - Reduces ammonia which is highly toxic to the central nervous system. Aspartic Acid may also increase resistance to fatigue and increase endurance.

TAURINE (Non-Essential Amino Acid) - Helps stabilize the excitability of membranes which is very important in the control of epileptic seizures. Taurine and sulfur are considered to be factors necessary for the control of many biochemical changes that take place in the aging process.

CYSTINE (Non-Essential Amino Acid) - Functions as an antioxidant and is a powerful aid to the body in protecting against radiation and pollution. It is necessary for the formation of the skin, which aids in the recovery from burns and surgical operations. Hair and skin are made up 10-14% Cystine.

HISTIDINE (Non-Essential Amino Acid) - Is found abundantly in hemoglobin; has been used in the treatment of rheumatoid arthritis, allergic diseases, ulcers & anemia. A deficiency can cause poor hearing.

PROLINE (Non-Essential Amino Acid) - Is extremely important for the proper functioning of joints and tendons, also helps maintain and strengthen heart muscles.

ALANINE (Non-Essential Amino Acid) - Is an important source of energy for muscle tissue, the brain and central nervous system, strengthens the immune system by producing antibodies and helps in the metabolism of sugars and organic acids.

For more, please visit: GlandularComplex.com

CHINESE MEDICINE AND HERBAL FORMULAS

Certainly herbs are turning heads these days as well. They contain phytochemicals store bought foods do not have which are said to heal us. This is why I offer Chinese Herbs and why shouldn't I?

Chinese herbs and chinese medicines have been used for thousands of years to help people feel better, more vital and live longer. Many of them have also been used for treating various illness and restoring the normal body functions for hundreds of years, and have proved their effectiveness. One of the most appealing qualities of Chinese herbs therapy is the low risk of adverse reaction or side effects, especially when compared to pharmaceutical drugs.

What's special about my Ultimate Herbal Formula? Alternative health care is under assault of mainstream medical corporations obsessed with profit-maximization by keeping you away from herbal remedies and on their drugs resulting in deceptive marketing and corruption of regulatory and educational institutions. To ethically serve and protect patients/clients from disinformation, we provide for you the defining qualities of the herbals in our formula.

Are these herbs Medicinal Herbs? The medicinal herbs info was compiled to help educate visitors about the often forgotten wisdom of the old ways of treating illnesses. Many of today's drugs and medicines were originally derived from natural ingredients, combinations of plants and other items found in nature. We are not suggesting that you ignore the help of trained medical professionals, simply that you have additional options available for treating illnesses. Often the most effective treatment involves a responsible blend of both modern and traditional treatments.

Is this Herbal Medicine: These products are unique, in that the ingredients are STANDARDIZED (i.e. their Bio-active substances are extracted under exacting standards to give each ingredient the highest possible full spectrum concentration). This unique process ensures that the products you buy are scientifically manufactured using the latest technology whilst retaining all the important natural ingredients.

Every ingredient is screened by qualified Botanists and subjected to Botanical and Chemical analysis. Thereafter they are processed in highly sophisticated equipment re-analysed to ensure they conform to rigid qualitative standards.

If you have used Don Lemmon's KNOW HOW products before then you already know the level of professionalism, the quality of his ingredients and the beauty of his presentations. This product contains a 30 day supply of capsules and each ingredient in Don Lemmon's Ultimate Herbal Formula has multiple benefits. Here are some very useful tid bits about all things it offers. Let's start with...

Chrysanthemum Flower (Ju Hua) - This flower of a special variety of Chrysanthemum is used in China to improve the circulation in the head and face and is thus traditionally used for headaches and sinus conditions. Since it has a cooling action, it is used to relieve red, swollen eyes such as that caused by smog and summer heat.

Mulberry Herb - It's availability of GABA lowers blood pressure, the phytosterol reduces cholesterol and deoxy-nojirimycin helps reducing blood sugar levels. Prevents you from a constipation without a laxative effect.

Dandelion Leaf - The root especially effects all forms of secretion and excretion from the body. By acting to remove poisons from the body, it acts as a tonic and stimulant as well.

Hawthorne Berry - European physicians often prescribe hawthorn as a substitute for digitalis, likely the most popular medicine for enhancing the contractility of a weakened heart.

Cocklebur Fruit - Opens the nasal passages, assists in dispersing breath, expels dampness, and relieves throat and nose itching.

Licorice Root - Helpful for gastric bleeding, prevention and for long term treatment of ulcers, and tissue rebuilding.

Angelica Root - Used to treat colds, indigestion, and rheumatism. The roots are liver and uterine stimulants.

Lycium Berry - A powerful antioxidant that contains 18 kinds of amino acids (six times higher than bee pollen), more beta carotene than carrots, and 500 times the amount of vitamin C by weight than oranges. It is loaded with vitamin B1, B2, B6 and Vitamin E. It has been found effective in increasing white blood cells, protecting liver function, lowering cholesterol, relieving hyper-tension, helping strengthen the immune system while building muscle tissue and burning body fat.

Suan Zao Seed - Nourishes and calms the heart and is a major traditional herb for insomnia.

Ginseng Root - Increases resistance to the effects of stress and improves circulation and mental functioning. Health conditions contributed to be stress include increased acidity of the body chemistry, back pain, cancer, Crohn's disease (inflammation of the intestinal tract), depression, chronic diarrhea, digestive disorders, hair loss, headaches, hypertension or high blood pressure, impotence, insomnia, TMJ syndromes (jaw pain and clicking), nervous and anxiety disorders, obsessive compulsive behaviors, various skin conditions, and finally, ulcers. Ginseng, whether it comes from Korea or Minnesota, is for people who have chronic fever, thirst, hot flashes, and crave sweets.

Chinese Asparagus Root - Chosen to strengthen the kidney and liver functions, improve vision and calm the nerves.

Walnut Fruit - Supports the digestive and glandular systems. Traditionally, black walnut hulls have been taken to enhance intestinal functioning, including soothing the lower intestinal tract and supporting the body's parasite-fighting efforts. Black Walnut is also high in iodine, and may help encourage glandular and thyroid health.

Longan Fruit - Used for the treatment of digestive problems, while Longan roots are known to promote the healing of bruises as well as breaking down phlegm for easier expulsion.

Codonopsis Root (Tang Shen) - Benefits the lungs and is helpful in treating chronic cough and shortness of breath.

Solomon's Seal Rhizome (Polyggonatum Multiflorum) - Rehydrates cells and prevents dehydration.

Dodder Seed - Dodder seed is considered to be a superior anti-aging herb and is used in vitality tonics to support the reproductive system.

Tangerine Peel - Regulates the digestion. Used for bloating, nausea and vomiting. Clears Phlegm.

Fo Ti Root - Can lower blood cholesterol levels, help prevent arteriosclerosis, reduce hypertension and lower incidence of coronary heart disease. Chinese medicine also indicates Fo-Ti as having anti-toxic, anti-swelling and tranquilizing properties as well as being useful for liver and spleen weakness, vertigo, scrofula, cancer, constipation and as a sedative for insomnia. Also recognized for having beneficial effects on fertility and other female functions involving ovulation.

Sesame Seed - Sesame seed benefits the body as a whole, especially the liver, kidney, spleen and stomach. Its high oil content lubricates the intestines and nourishes all the internal viscera. It also blackens one's hair, especially the black sesame. Hence, it is applied to white hair, habitual constipation, and insufficient lactation. Sesame oil is also helpful in treating intestinal worms like ascaris, tapeworm, etc.

Ligustrum Fruit - Boosts immunity and relieves stress.

Eclipta Herb - Used as a rejuvenative herb which supports the mind, nerves, eyes and hair. It is also traditionally used for liver disorders in both systems of medicine. Modern research has shown that in some ways certain constituents of Eclipta are superior to those of Milk Thistle in the protection of liver cells.

Cherokee Rose Fruit - A sour, cherry-like fruit that binds and contains the body's energies thus preserving resistant function.

Siegesbeckia Herb - In China it is used as a remedy for ague, rheumatism, and renal colic, used in Britain chiefly as a cure for ringworm in conjunction with glycerine and used in Mauritius Islands for syphilis, leprosy, and various skin diseases.

Eucommia Bark - A superb Yang Jing herb, used to strengthen the back (especially the lower back), skeleton, and joints (especially the knees and ankles). Eucommia is believed to confer strength and flexibility to the ligaments and tendons.

Ox Knee Root - Promotes blood circulation to regulate menstruation, nourishes the liver and kidneys, strengthens bones and muscles, induces diuresis to cure strangury (a painful discharge of urine, drop by drop) and conducts fire (blood) downward.

Honeysuckle Vine - Anti-inflammatory herb.

Sheng Di Root - Nourishes joints, tendons, ligaments and muscle.

Schisandra Fruit - Traditionally used for exhaustion, low libido, insomnia, and liver problems. In Chinese medicine they are also used to strengthen the kidneys and restore the fluid balance in the body.

Cistanche Root - To moisten the intestines and warm the womb.

China Root - Benefits spleen and for bloody dysentery.

Sweetflag Rhizome - It is widely employed in modern herbal medicine as an aromatic stimulant and mild tonic. In Ayurveda it is highly valued as a rejuvenator for the brain and nervous system and as a remedy for digestive disorders.

Anise Seed (Pimpinnella Anisum) - Used for flatulence, indigestion, infant colic, hiccup, coughs and bronchial catarrh.

Dipsacus Root - Strengthens the spleen and dries excessive internal dampness.

Chinese Senega Root - Support for relief of stress and nervous irritability.

Chinese Yam Root - Wild yam root has been used for hundreds of years to treat rheumatism and arthritis-like ailments. The discovery of steroidal glycosides (diosgenin) in the root validated this ancient practice.

Gui Yuan (Longan) - Regulates appetite, stimulates gastric juices and improves bowel function.

Lotus Seed (Sm Nelumbinis) - A mild sedative useful for alleviating nervousness and irritability.

Qian Shi Fruit (Sm Euryales) - Strengthens the spleen and kidneys respectively and relieves chronic loose stool that is a result of weakness in these organs.

Coicis Seed (Pearl Barley - Job's Tears) - It enters the spleen, stomach, lungs and large intestine to tonify these organs.

Echinacea Angustifolia (Angustifolia Root Extract) - First used by Native Americans as a remedy for skin wounds and snakebites. Today, the herb is highly regarded for its benefits in strengthening the immune system. Studies show echinacea to even help treat conditions like psoriasis and eczema.

Iris Versicolor Extract (Blue Flag Root Extract) - The protector of the thymus gland, controller of immunity.

Hydrastis Canadensis (Golden Seal Root Extract) - This herb contains berberine and other natural compounds having numerous health benefits. Taken at the first signs of respiratory problems, colds or flu, Goldenseal can help prevent further symptoms from developing.

Alfalfa - It is often used to aid digestion, help heal bone disorders and is often recommended as an anti-inflammatory.

Bee Pollen - Hailed as a cure all but one interesting point is that of the 28 minerals in the human body, most are considered essential. Bee pollen contains all 28 minerals...

Black Radish Root (Raphanus Sativus) - Black Radish is rich in vitamin C, which helps us fight infections and free radicals. Black radish also contains a variety of chemicals that increase the flow of bile which play an important role in the digestion process. Radish help maintain a healthy gallbladder. It also has an antibacterial effect on our digestive flora.

Dandelion Root (Taraxacum Officinale) - For centuries, dandelion root has been regarded as an effective, gentle laxative. The roots and leaves are used to treat liver conditions and to encourage normal digestion. All parts of the plant have high concentrations of vitamin A, and choline, a B vitamin that stimulates the liver.

Siberian Ginseng (Eleuthero Root) - Siberian Ginseng Strengthens the adrenal and reproductive glands. Enhances immune function, promotes lung functioning and stimulates the appetite. Useful for bronchitis, circulatory problems, diabetes, infertility, lack of energy, and stress. Said to help ease withdrawl from cocaine, and to protect against the effects of radiation exposure. Used by athletes for overall body strengthening. May help improve drug or alcohol induced liver dysfunction in older adults.

Fringe Tree Root (Chionanthus Virginicus) - It is renown for their tonic effect on the liver and digestive system.

Garlic - Garlic helps to prevent cancer. It prevents the further growth of certain tumors while reducing the size of others.

Gentian Root (Gentiana Lutea) - For the pancreas, digestive organs, kidney, spleen, glands, jaundice and liver disorders.

Gota Kola - Brain food, memory, depression, vitality, senility.

Greater Celandine Herb (Chelidonium Majus) - Used to treat conditions of the liver and other conditions.

Green Beet Leaf (Beta Vulgaris) - Provide liver support for normal fat metabolism.

Green Pea Concentrate - Provides support for cardiovascular health.

Hawthorn Berry (Crataegus Oxyacantha) - It helps to increase the utilization of oxygen in the heart while increasing enzyme metabolism in the heart muscle.

Kola Nut - Good for sinus, phlegm, arthritis and strengthens the immune system. Helps the nervous system and increases brain power.

Korean Ginseng - This famously energizing herb has been found to improve abstract thinking, speed up reaction time, and boost resistance to viral infections.

Milk Thistle (Seed) - Milk thistle is a potent anti-oxidant, more potent than Vitamins C and E. This means it can counteract free radical damage that can cause degenerative diseases including cancer.

Muira Puama - Used for sex, menstrual cramps and PMS, and central nervous system disorders.

Nettles Leaf (Urtica Dioica) - In addition to its ability to have antihistamine-like effect, nettles tonify and firm inflamed tissues.

Parsley Leaf (Petroselinum Crispun) - Effective diuretic, also aids menstruation and eases colic pains.

Saw Palmetto Berries - Saw Palmetto is often mislabeled as a man's herb. While it certainly has many benefits on the prostate for men, it holds an important place in this formula for women. Traditionally considered a uterine tonic, long been used for painful menstruation, and ovarian pain and inflammation.

Yellow Dock - Stimulates liver bile, clear toxins, and are used for chronic skin disorders. They treat psoriasis and constipation.

Water Plantain Root - It supplements the spleen, benefits energy, converts excessive moisture, and promotes diuresis.

Shou Di Root (Rhemenia Root) - Helps in promoting blood circulation and improvement in vital energy.

Mint Leaf - An antioxidant that cleans the skin.

Cassia Tora Seed - Known for helping to lower blood cholesterol, uric acids and sugar levels, reduce kidney and gall stones, improve digestion, normalize blood pressure and dissolve blood clots.

Amazing, isn't it? Just how did we fit so many nutrients in one capsule and allow just 6 capsules a day to be enough to benefit you? Because we have combined specific ingredients in specific dosages that work hand in hand together like a team with no fillers, binders, or any other fluff other companies are giving you. The search for the fountain of youth has continued throughout the ages. It would be great if there existed a pill derived from natural sources to insure a long and healthy life, but no such magical pill exists. In the meantime, the best solution is to take impeccable care of ourselves. There really is no other way around it but there are things now in pill form that help. Taking excellent care of ourselves requires a multitude of lifestyle decisions including, but not limited to, nutrition, exercise, stress, sex, emotions, and rest. So much to learn, so much to do, so many decisions to make in such a short time. Just knowing where to begin on this self-care quest can present a dilemma, not to mention the challenge of making the right health choices on a continuing basis once you actually decide what they are.

Let us help you make a choice. If you are ready to try a full month supply of this Ultimate Herbal Formula (180 capsules), simply drop me an email or visit UltimateHerbalFormula.com today! This product, along with our Glandular Complex have been the products all diets have been missing for far too long. The herbs alone are normally $20 and the glands $30. But through this book, both are being made available to you for just $39.95 a month! Contact us today to place your order!

THE PROTEIN POWDER AND MEAL REPLACEMENT FAD

I gave up on meal replacements almost as soon as they hit the market. Sure, every time a new one came out claiming to be nothing like the last, I fell for it, but not since 1994 have I found one that at least had natural ingredients. I realize protein supplements are one of the most popular food supplements available and that many of you believe you will deflate, get fat or the earth will stop spinning if you aren't using them but listen up.

Although meal replacements (bars or shakes) provide carbohydrate, protein and some fat, these supplements have a deserved but hush-hush bad reputation because they also contain artificial colors, sweeteners, corn syrup, hydrogenated oils, modified starches and other ingredients which are the same things in candy and cake mix. I couldn't take it any longer and had my own created. I call it the Complete Protein Powder.

What we have here is plain, bland, no frills and complete protein powder that really is special. In fact, I challenge you to compare it to anything else on the market. Our secret is the precise ratio blend of whey, rice and soy proteins and the purity and no genetically modified sources. We refused to use the cheaper ingredients like the popular hydrolized contents, tar, ash, etc, nor the other hidden fillers that you read about which are otherwise bad for you despite the sales claims.

This powder is so clean that you can forget about needing a whole cup to attain 25 grams of protein. We give you that in just about 3 regular sized tablespoons. How so? It's because there is nothing in there we failed to list like corn starch many companies haven't told you about. What about your meal replacements? Isn't this just protein powder? Yes, but mix it in ice water with a TB of Lemmon's Oil and you have a complete meal. Take your multi-vitamin, herbs, glands and you cannot find a more complete snack.

Protein supplements are now and will probably always one of the most popular food supplements available. Along the same lines, meal replacement supplements such as MET-Rx® or Slim-Fast® are recommended to be eaten in place of several meals. The main benefit they supposedly offer is one of convenience, together with a controlled portion size. Compare a typical 250 calorie meal replacement supplement to a giant bowl of cereal or a king-size hamburger and you'll realize they're a very easy way to slash hundreds of calories from your diet but do they nourish you? The problem comes when deciding which product you should use but it is as simple as reading the label. Magazines aren't really much help. They float on advertising dollars and are reluctant to print anything that will discourage potential advertisers especially when the advertiser and the magazine are one and the same people!

In regards to our using soy, though soy proteins contain estrogenic compounds, it appears that they are tissue and sex specific. Several studies found that soy proteins, unaltered, not genetically modified and all natural, had no effects on the reproductive hormones of men and balanced those in women. All the measures you could imagine were taken.

Furthermore, the scientists found no difference between male animals who ate soy protein that contained the plant estrogens and those who ate soy with the estrogens removed, leading researchers to conclude isoflavones do improve cardiovascular risk factors without apparent deleterious effects on the male reproductive system...

I like everyone else can appreciate a good protein powder. The problem is, with all the protein powders on the market, what is the best? Everyone claims to have "The Best Whey Protein" but how can they? It's either pure or it's not... It is either filler free or it's not...

I also realize pure protein powder is tasteless and if anything you will need soy protein powder recipes just to get the stuff down and I also understand that the whey protein powder recipes listed on the labels are great but they aren't great for you...

Either way, yes, there are literally dozens of different of supposedly complex and complete proteins, pure proteins and other protein powders on the market. The questions I am most often presented are: What is the best? Where do you get it? How much do you need? Is it necessary? How do you use it? Where can you get it without added fillers and binders and junk?

Quote: "This is actually the only protein currently on the market that we've seen to work with cream to actually increase muscularity and lower body fat. Others tend to cause a slight decrease in vascularity and definition. It is not the cream. Protein and fat belong side by side. It is your choice of protein." Have you heard this before only to buy something that ends up sending you on a sugar fit or makes you fat?

Me too... You're not alone... I am not against popping amino acids tablets or taking additional glutamine at times (glutamine builds your immunity as it is the most abundant of the aminos necessary) but these companies aren't selling you what they are hyping to you....

You are better off with more protein than wasting money on what's in your foods... We certainly do require a dozen different essential amino acids available at each protein meal if we want results... This is the only other food deficiency supplementation can eliminate besides vitamins and minerals (found in our Perfect Vitamin) and essential fatty acids (found in our Lemmon's Oil). It is well known that BCAA (branch chain amino acids found in our Glandular Complex) are the building blocks of all the other amino acids and comprise over a third of your muscle tissue...

So why not just supplement with those? A great deal of the BCAA our body has in store from your diet is lost during exercise (they are L-Leucine, L-Isoleucine, and L-Valine) so just maybe..... I would say just to use powders as long as you're not depending upon them as your only protein source because when you are tired of food, there still isn't a need to stress the body into turning one nutrient into another nor limiting it of the things it needs to assist the process. We need complete proteins to do the job right.

Remember, if it smells or tastes like cake batter, IT USUALLY IS. Iso-this, ultra pure-that, and all the tricks the fitness companies are trying to seduce you are amazing.

3 tablespoons of our truly pure protein contains 25 grams of protein, a couple carbs and only a gram or two of fat. What else is in the health food containers that you need 6 tablespoons for the same amount of protein? Mystery meat?

I can mix the protein I sell in peanut butter. In fact, we here love my special mix of almond butter, peanut butter, sesame butter, Lemmon's Oil and just enough powder to equal a 3 to 1 ratio of protein to fat.

Persons with kidney stones may benefit from this product but keep in mind all protein supplements should be pure and 100% nothing but protein or what is found in the source naturally to work for and not against you.

Never allow for added fillers or binders or other junk you do not need. Proteins are naturally carbohydrate free for the most part and will always contain a little fat. But sugar? Never.

Do yourself a favor, throw out all protein powders and meal replacements or lo-carb bars right now.

They are nothing more than corn syrup, milk powder, b-complex vitamins and lard. If you want real success, you should eat real food and try what I am talking about here. Our Complete Protein Powder contains certain globulin proteins which inhibit unhealthy bacteria from attaching to your intestinal walls, but is still only meant to be a supplement to REAL food. You're looking for results, right?

Well one thing's for certain... No matter how hard you train... No matter what supplements you take.... To build new muscle you need protein.... The better the protein... The better the results... And you need to provide your muscles with the nutrients to repair, rebuild, and grow... Every moment of every day!

How much protein is it you need? How often do you ingest it? How many times have you heard the statement, "You can get all the protein you need from a normal diet?" The question is, "Need for what? And what is normal? Who are they kidding?"

There's quite a difference between the need to sustain life, rebuild health and the need to achieve a premium muscular body. To sustain life they say you need about 36 grams of protein per 100 lb. of bodyweight. I say that's enough if you lay on your back without blinking each day...

To regenerate health you may want to supplement this much more to the diet in our Complete Protein Powder form... To build muscle however... Recent research has shown three times this amount may be required to obtain maximum increases in strength and lean mass in less than 30 days....

See for yourself. Try doubling your protein intake with for a few days, then add our product and watch what happens! It only takes a matter of days to notice a big difference in terms of muscularity and strength. Increasing your complete protein intake almost always results in greater muscularity.

This maxes out the amino acid content of the muscles, giving them a harder, fuller appearance. Your hormonal system also gets involved, switching over from fat storing to a fat burning mode through the release of the hormone glucagon. This fat burning hormone is released in response to a greater protein to essential fat (found in our Lemmon's Oil) ratio in your diet. Sure, to achieve this, you could simply lower carbohydrates and increase fat, but you'd lose a lot of muscle.

If anything we have discussed is your goal, increase your protein intake to having 1/3 your lean mass amount in grams four times a day, you cannot fail. No one EVER has. That would be 60 grams 4 times a day for someone with 180 pounds of lean mass.

Can you ingest 240 grams of protein a day without supplements? Sure, but it's a lot easier to eat three major food meals and two or three minor ones, supplementing or replacing the minor ones with a delicious milkshake and a complete multi-vitamins and mineral (found in our Balanced Multi-Nutrient).

One of the easiest, yet most neglected ways to use our complete protein powder is to take it right along with your existing protein meals. Not only will it increase your total protein intake, but the high amounts of essential amino acids will complete the amino profile of your whole food sources giving you even greater protein utilization for sure fire results.

Is this too much protein at one time? Only if you want to stay small, weak or unhealthy! You'll never get anywhere ignoring this information.

I mix 2/3 with ice water and 1 tb of lemmons oil 2 times a day in a blender with about 12 oz water..... I also eat 6 food meals....

If you want to get yourself a 2 pound jar with 30 servings for only $19.95, please visit www.CompleteProteinPowder.com

DRINKING ENOUGH WATER

If you feel that you are retaining water even though you drink water all day long, or if you rarely go to the bathroom then you probably SIP water all day and don't realize you have to CHUG it. If that's what you do and you're still bloating and not peeing, you had better rush to a doctor. That's not right. Since the odds are more likely that you are dehydrated, I suggest doubling your water intake and adding more fiber to the diet.

Besides everything else we have discussed, by far the most important thing the human body requires next to air is water. Water makes up the largest overall percentage of our physical being (muscles alone are comprised of over 2/3 H2O). It regulates numerous functions which otherwise slow down without it like maintaining the elasticity of your skin, eliminating wrinkles, lubricating joints, balancing blood volume, controlling the ability to attack viruses, getting rid of constipation, urinary tract issues and generally everything else from sleeping to thinking.

With this in mind, you should try to drink a gallon of filtered, purified or distilled water for every 100 pounds you weigh each and every day in order to provide yourself with a proper level of hydration. This amount of fluid will suffice in eliminating the urge to drink coffee, tea, fat producing juices, sodas and other liquids that you really don't need. If you do drink one of these other liquids, don't worry yourself over it, just be sure to have an extra equal amount of fresh clean water to wash it down.

You need to go pee-pee as often as possible the first couple of weeks. By then, your bladder will adjust to the new routine. This is important to know because every time you pee the body excretes toxins and flushes your fat right down the toilet! So, drink enough at all times to keep your urine clear. Letting it turn yellow is a sure sign of a set back.

Water should be drank upon waking, 15 minutes after each meal, between each meal, before, after, and during workouts, before bed and then again at all other times you feel thirsty. That is approximately a dozen minimum daily servings. A gallon of water has 128 ounces. Divided by 12 that is only 10 ounces of water 12 times a day for each gallon you are to complete by day's end.

If you are required a gallon and a half, that would be 15 ounces 12 times a day. For 2 gallons, have 20 ounces at a time. I weigh around 200 pounds but am pretty active and I currently live in the desert (Las Vegas, Nevada) so I personally keep a 24-ounce cup full of water by my side or on my desk at all times. You should drink water throughout the day, even if you wake up in the middle of the night. Especially if you wake up with muck (dry) mouth.

Drinking water at night or in the morning before getting up through a straw (still laying down) is a good thing because your valves stay open while lying down and that allows for a faster quenching of all your tissues. As we grow older, our thirst mechanism is less efficient. We sometimes have to remind ourselves to drink. So always have that glass, cup, jug or bottle handy and full of fresh water to keep yourself reminded. The glasses of water you drink between meals should be cold if possible. If you are obese, make that water not just with ice in them but actually ICE COLD.

The internal cooling effect the ice initiates inside of you will speed the metabolism up (to warm you) and you'll burn more calories. When I say ice water, I do not mean you should be sitting around sucking or eating cubes. If you have this habit, it could stem from what is known as pagophagia. It is a disorder that is commonly associated with iron deficiency anemia. You probably have other cravings for food and some non-food items too. Do you also chew your ink pens and fingernails? This is relevant in 50% of such patients with a mineral deficiency.

That's all it is. Luckily over 70 different minerals that your body requires is in my Multi-Nutrient Formula. If you do not like the taste of water, in time, you will, but for now, add some fresh lemon or apple cider vinegar to it (especially if you have a cold as this kills bad bacteria). I get my apple cider vinegar from Omega Nutrition. It's made the old fashioned way which leaves all the vitamins, minerals, amino acids, pectin, fiber, healthy bacteria and enzymes intact.

Be certain you only have this cold water with cider or lemon juice in it BETWEEN meals because the acids could destroy your digestive enzymes. They boost your enzymes if you use them between, but during, no way. And make sure you get the cider from Omega. Regular old store bought isn't good enough.

As far as the water drank with or after meals, it should be room temperature and SIPPED, not chugged or gulped, if drank at all, during the meal. Having 4 to 8 ounces sipped at a meal is fine, that doesn't hurt. But drinking a lot of water to 'wash' your food down mid meal is not a good idea. If you do not pay attention to these things, you will have trouble digesting your foods, let alone flushing nitrogenous waste, toxins, body fat and even poo-poo out on a 'regular' basis. Just remember, if you dehydrate, kidney function is tweaked, waste products accumulate, and the body's sole reaction is to retain all the water it has left. You will bloat and until you get enough water back in the system, your engine cannot become healthy again. The liver will certainly try anyhow (stressing itself out) attempting to flush out the excess waste on it's own.

As a result, fat burning is shut down and you become fatigued, bloated, aggravated at the drop of a dime and did I mention migraines? Oh, you already get them? I wonder why... Next, I suggest getting a home water filtration product of some sort. You may get by without it, and you may think your tap water is alright, but in most cases, fish would die if left alone in the average glass or tank of plain old tap water.

Trust me, if a gold fish can't survive in tap water, it can't be good for you either. Don't stop there. I want you to get a good shower filter too. You are what you absorb and everything you are trying to avoid by drinking only purified water will still get absorbed (through your skin) while bathing anyhow.

Hey, you are washing in tap water. You don't have to drink it to absorb the chemicals in it so be careful. Tap water contains chlorine, which destroys the healthy bacteria in your gut, and that is what makes illness difficult to deal with. This is also why I said that when you buy your water, you should shoot for distilled water. I do not trust what is in spring water nor what is in most grocery store bought drinking water either. Many brands are nothing more than filtered tap water, which is sometimes fine, but it's not boiled of all impurities like distilled.

Here you thought you knew all there was to know about water.

So, let's recap.

If you weigh 100 pounds, drink one full gallon a day (128 ounces).

If you weigh 125 pounds, have one and one quarter gallon a day (160 ounces).

If you weigh 150 pounds, have one and one half gallon (192 ounces).

175 pounds a day requires one and three quarters gallon (224 ounces).

If you weigh 200 pounds, that's 2 gallons a day and so on and so on. Yes, if you weigh 300 pounds, I expect you to drink 3 gallons of water NOT SODA between waking up and going back to sleep each day. This is hardly a lot to ask!

ARTIFICIAL SWEETENERS

I don't care how bland you feel your food is, there is nothing wrong with the way natural foods taste. Thinking you need artificial flavoring on everything is a sure sign of how chemically dependant you've become. I have had many clients who abused their intake of artificial sweeteners to a point they needed medical attention. Do you really want it to go that far? One woman I used to know in particular ate 120 packets of artificial sweeteners a day. Yeah, 120. And her withdrawal symptoms were horrifying. Things like nutra-sweet, aspartame, sucralose, splenda and saccharine are not natural foodstuffs. They are chemicals.

They are drugs. Drugs, that when their temperature exceeds room temperature, like inside the body or a cup of coffee, converts these wood alcohols into formaldehyde and formic acid. You know what that is. Formic acid is the same poison found in insects like fire ants and scorpions. Sure, not as much, but enough to cause metabolic acidosis and methanol toxicity that gives innocent victims symptoms of multiple sclerosis. I have been given reports of people suddenly beginning ['to']tremble, becoming blurry eyed and even hearing bells in their ears after drinking diet soda.

If you suffer from any disease symptoms such as spasms, joint or organ pains, numbness in your limbs, cramps in your muscles, sudden dizziness, headaches, depression, anxiety, slurred speech, or memory loss and you are using chemical sweeteners, then you need to stop whether you think it is related or not. The memory loss is due to the aspartic acid used to make these sweeteners. It goes past the blood brain barrier and deteriorates your neurons eventually causing seizures. The phenylalanine used to make these sweeteners is mutated so it depletes serotonin, causes manic depression, panic attacks, rage and violence in otherwise calm, cool and collected individuals.

I realize the sugar industry has added artificial sweeteners to our foods but relabeled those foods as healthier alternatives but if they aren't harmful to begin with, how can you label something as healthier or SAFER? Something is either healthy and safe or it isn't. If you say SAFER, are you implying that before, it wasn't safe enough? Sounds fishy to me. I honestly feel nothing can be done to stop the distribution of these chemicals in our foods but we can refuse to buy or eat anything that contains them.

That's a great place to start. I personally stopped drinking decaf coffee once I found out the industry uses bleaches and formaldehyde to remove the caffeine. I am not a caffeine junky, but I do like my occasional coffee and once I began to avoid the formaldehyde, man, my health did a complete turn around. I couldn't figure out why, even though it was decaf, I still got the jitters. Have you ever drank a cup of decaf and suffered a little 'night' blindness in the middle of the afternoon? That was the formaldehyde poisoning your retina.

The methanol in your artificial sweeteners converts to formaldehyde. Formaldehyde is just like cyanide and arsenic. It attacks nerve endings, changes body chemistry and causes neurological disorders even when taking the smallest amounts. I used to tell people to just limit their intake but now that I know and have experienced the difference myself, I demand you stop using them immediately. If for no other reason, stop using artificial sweeteners because they are also part of the reason you crave carbohydrates. Do you remember what happens to extra carbs? It becomes hard to reach body fat. What do carbs mixed with chemicals become? Cellulite.

And any formaldehyde that hasn't damaged you yet, will, because it is stored in your fat cells, particularly those in the hip and thigh areas. Yummy. Do you like carrying around grotesque, jello-looking, bouncing, cellulite? This is also another reason why when you start to lose fat on this program that you feel so nasty and crabby.

Your fat cells are dumping out all those stored chemicals for excretion. Live with it because sooner or later, you won't have that choice unless you rid yourself of this gunk as soon as possible.

And trust me, the manufacturers of these poisons know how awful for you they are. Their funding/lobbying of the American Diabetes Association, American Dietetic Association, Congress and even the American medical associations is nothing more than blood money. So, what's the solution for a sweet tooth? Besides trying to just get used to the natural flavors of food, there is always stevia. Stevia is a natural herb and food sweetener, which also helps in the metabolism of sugar as opposed to tricking your body into thinking it too is a carbohydrate. That's what these artificial sweeteners do. They trick your body into thinking it's getting sugar so you'll still suffer from insulin woes on top of everything else.

From now on, if it says "sugar free" "no sugar added" or "dietetic" on the food label, check for what chemicals it contains before buying it! Even if it says "fat free" or "nonfat" still read the label. Companies like EAS and Met-rx are poisoning you with artificial sweeteners, hydrogenated oils and cheap ingredients. You do not even realize it nor do they care. Most people may think modern medicine has all the answers but the latest medical research is released daily that proves the marketing hype to sell artificial sweeteners wrong. You know it, I know and it's time everyone else knows it. Spread the word. You'll thank me one day.

Friends don't let friends drink diet soda, use protein powders or eat foods that contain artificial sweeteners. I had a decaf coffee recently that I was told happened to be a naturally caffeine free blend. I was also told the creamer in the container was real cream, not artificial. I didn't have 3 sips before my speech slurred, my vision blurred and my head pounded.

It took a 3 hour nap to recover. All chemicals are poisons. Mix them with hydrogenated oils and you're killing yourself.

When I say I do not know a single athlete, model or bodybuilder that has more than one meal replacement shake a day, I mean it. In fact, I had a rather well known spokes model for one best selling protein powder brands on the market announce on my radio show that most of the before and after pictures her former company used were fakes. Another mutual friend has endorsed a particular line found in grocery stores for the past 5 years says she cannot use the stuff at all. It gives her hives! What's in that crap? Crap.

What I have presented so far is merely what I have personally discovered in research, school, counsel, at seminars, and etc. I met a man named Dr Gary Eversole who taught me about a missing link I never before considered back in 1993 through a mutual friend who was being treated by him. This friend came to me one day and said he had a doctor that was doing all these amazing things for him without the use of drugs.

Well, I put it off but finally went in to see him a few weeks later and much to my surprise, this was a real doctor after all. I hadn't seen one for a while and this guy seemed confident he could teach me something that could alleviate my current issues. Always being willing to learn and knowing he simply wanted to exchange services, I went along with it. What I knew about anatomy and everyday 'normal' things we commonly do to remain healthy changed in a matter of 20 minutes. You could assume I discovered I was toxic and required an overhaul, oil change, tune up and having my pipes cleaned but it was more enlightening than that. Dr Gary Eversole taught me in 20 minutes that health was within our grasp and we can call all our own shots. He is a REAL doctor, not some sort of homeopath, and I would rather he speak for himself. Here he is.

ALTERNATIVE HEALTH CARE

Hi! I am Dr. Gary Eversole! Did you know that nagging pain, which afflicts us all on one occasion or another, has a deeper affect upon your health than just causing us to hunch over in agony? This chapter is all about how arthritis or an old football injury may just be one or two steps away from causing you to become cancerous. Do I have your attention? Well, those pains are also the difference between success and failure in fat loss and building muscle too. So pay attention. Generally, eighty percent of the population will suffer from muscular or joint pain at one time or another, and it is currently the number one reason people go to the emergency room.

Billions of dollars are spent annually by those of you seeking relief so some one is aching. In fact, one in three people have pain in their neck or back ALL the time. That's the most feared ailment of man. Rightly so, an aching back leads to almost every other ailment and disease we can name. It's something that needs taken care of as soon as it arises. As a practicing physician, I have come to the realization that drugs and surgery are useless, for the most part, in helping you live without pain. In fact, more than three fourths of all back surgeries fail and at best, drugs only cover up the pain you have for a short period of time.

I have worked on many surgical disasters that came into my office and have gotten even more people to stop taking unnecessary medications. The truth is, the only way you can effectively eliminate joint pain, especially in the low back is to make some lifestyle changes. Those changes are both mental and physical. My point is not to make you or your medical doctors sound like they are evil or hiding the truth about this matter from you. In most cases, like with nutrition, most physicians aren't taught what I am going to explain to you today. It's all very simple and easy to understand.

I know you will enjoy what I have in store for you. Over the years, my patients have come up with many reasons for why they think they have acquired their aches and pains but rarely is it from what they think. The list of reasons why a person's different parts supposedly hurt is endless, and while many things they think may have in fact caused one or two body parts to start hurting, it is usually the 'last' straw, the one that broke the camel's back (or my patient's back) so to speak that ails you! What I'm trying to say here is that people do little things over days, months, or years, and in time, just like adding one more straw, little by little, more and more to some poor camel's back, also causes your spine to break little by little too.

A good healthy back does not fall apart all at once, folks. It is weakened over time by many of the very everyday things we do without even realizing it. Once the back goes, on comes the pain for the other joints, muscles and organs. What are the things we do everyday to weaken or damage our low backs? They are: stresses (of all sorts), exposure to toxins (both drugs, environmental and other poisons), plus physical trauma (brought on by accidental and intentional outside forces). There are two major types of stress that affect our bodies mental and physical. Mental stress occurs when we allow our emotions to get out of control and get the best of us.

Destructive emotions such as worry, fear, hate and anger, are sources of mental stress. Overwhelming challenges in our lives such as bills, raising children, and driving to work may also cause mental stress but we both know we sometimes make matters worse than they need to be. Do you make mountains out of mole hills? Are you someone who likes to email others in fits of rage but realize afterwards the other person really hadn't done anything to make you act that way? It's just stress and it's all something we must learn to control. Physical stress occurs when outside forces act on our bodies.

Examples of this would be things that happen because we are over-working, poorly conditioned due to lack of exercise, exposed to extreme weather conditions, or when something causes us physical injuries (which we will cover under the topic of trauma). Some mental and physical stress is good as it motivates us to do something about situations that we don't want to be in, or we may even learn to solve a problem that makes us more comfortable in future situations. These kinds of stress are the ones they say make us stronger.

However, too much of a good thing is harmful. Even too much exercise is stressful. When we are under stress, interesting changes occur inside our bodies. The body responds to stress first by causing the adrenal gland, which is located just above the kidney, to produce and secrete an increased amount of 'stress' hormones, which then circulate into the body via the bloodstream (like cortisol). This increased amount of adrenal hormone is what gets our bodies ready for ACTION by increasing our metabolic rate. It causes that 'excited' feeling we all get when scared. However, your metabolic rate is the measurement of the speed at which our body uses up its nutrients, or fuels.

Things we desperately need when we are performing other mental or physical functions. These nutrients, or body fuels, which come from the foods we eat, the supplements we take and even the water we drink are supposed to do other things besides get burnt up when we stress ourselves out. When the metabolic rate is increased because of stress, our bodies use up our nutrients at such an increased rate, sometimes it does not leave any extra nutrients available so that our bodies can even come close to handling the stress. As you use up your nutrients, you will first start to become tired and fatigued.

When we deplete in such a manner, obviously, we need replenishment. But that is only part of the picture. Every one of us, at some point in our lives, has experienced a situation that really frightened us.

Like the time you were almost in a car accident, or caught in a lie, the time you thought you had lost a child or a parent, or the time you walked into that dark house and your friend jumped out of a dark corner and yelled, "BOO!" Afterwards, you found yourself shaking all over, feeling weak, and possibly even like you were going to be sick. Stress like this is extremely harmful to all of the body's systems, so you can imagine what trouble lies ahead if this type of stress occurs every day, month after month, and year after year and you do nothing to 'replenish' yourself!

It can lead to an extremely weak, troubled and worn out body. This type of body is susceptible to damage from physical stresses, especially in the areas of its main frame and support structure, the back. Whenever the spine is affected, eventually, so is your overall health. You see, our backs are made up of bones called vertebrae that have plates between them called discs. At the bottom of this stack of vertebrae and discs is an area of the lower back called the lumbar spine. It is held together, much like the rest of the spine, by soft tissue called muscle and ligaments. Sounds like the rest of the body actually, doesn't it.

Well, the difference is, when our bodies get into a state of fatigue due to stress, the nutrients depleted leave these particular muscles and ligaments in a fatigued state too. They're the first to go. The next problem arises once these muscles loosen up. It's almost like they 'give' up all at once but in reality they have been going through stresses of their own after trying so hard for so long to keep things from falling apart. However, since you continued to work against the muscle's original plan (holding you together), eventually things have to fail. You don't eat right, you don't take your supplements, you don't exercise, you don't... You don't get the picture. Do all you can to relax and take care of yourself from now on or... You might first feel it when you do certain things repeatedly, such as bending over for groceries, sleeping in certain positions, or sitting for prolonged periods of time.

All it takes is for you to perform a movement one day that we all do on a regular basis and think nothing of it. However, when we are in a state of fatigue or depletion, anything we do, no matter how normal it supposedly is, may be that last thing we remembered which damaged our low backs. Stress is unavoidable.

Making mountains out of mole-hills is your own doing. Due to not only your previous stresses but also the bad posture you have adopted since the lower back made it's changes, things only get worse. What happens next occurs when the joints between the vertebrae, which contain your discs, become overtaxed or worn out. The vertebrae will now slip from their normal positions creating a push and pull situation between your delicate discs. Picture it. What you have is a vertebrae sliding to the left and becoming slack but over on the right, your ligaments are pulling and pulling trying to get it back in place. What happens if now they give up too and loosen like the lower back did? It affects the rest of your nervous system.

Your vertebrae and discs form holes where they meet on both the left and right side of the spine. These holes are where spinal nerves come through from the spinal cord. The spinal cord then connects to all of the nerves of the body this way, each therefore directly attached to the brain in your head and supposedly protected by the vertebrae.

But when the vertebrae slips out of position, it affects the size of the hole that the nerve comes out of. This affects that particular nerve adversely as the relationship between those nerves, the spinal chord and your brain will not be whole. We may not feel any pain at first, not even when the lower back gives out, which is usually the case, but the damage is done anyhow, silently, and that damage adds up little by little. Eventually, you feel it. Oh, you will feel it. It may not be for months or even years that we have back pain, but when it finally manifests itself, now you know, it means something has been wrong for awhile.

And this is just the beginning. Your pain means those nerves inside of you aren't doing their jobs and many other systems of the body are headed for trouble. Toxins are the second biggest factor that affects this process and they are any substance that causes a chemical change in the body. Toxins are air pollutants, pesticides on our foods, the drugs we keep around our homes, caffeine, alcohol, artificial sweeteners and things that aren't supposed to be in our tap water, but are. Sure, we can control some of these things, like the air we breathe can be made better if we move out of the city, but in many cases water is a problem everywhere.

Let's just focus on drugs. Prescription, non-prescription, narcotics, pharmaceuticals, recreational, sports related, or whatever you're taking to ease the pain. Drugs are another silent killer. I say this because drugs are accepted and widely used, even revered by our society but drugs are only meant for temporary use. Your little pills and shots only make temporarily UN-natural chemical changes in our bodies to merely rid our body of its symptoms, not the disease. They were never meant to be a cure. Drug commercials on television even say they are for temporary relief.

They also mention that list of side effects a mile long). Really? Of course they do. So here is what can happen when you take those pharmaceutical goodies:

1) Your bodies become dependent of the drugs and stops producing its own chemicals which relieve the same symptoms naturally or...

2) The drugs destroy essential nutrients and hormones in our bodies, causing low energy, fatigue and even dis-ease. Our bodies really do have their own abilities to beat pain and we recognize drugs as toxins once they get inside of us. That's just another stress you really won't need at this point.

So, besides stress, if we take drugs to get rid of our symptoms, then our bodies will stop relying on their own abilities. Hence, the rule applies, "If you don't use it, you lose it!" I know sometimes pain can be unbearable. But once you deal with the cause of the pain, it will disappear. Just imagine for a second what is going on inside of you when you are experiencing stress AND using drugs at the same time once your nerves become impaired. The impact on your health would be extremely detrimental.

You are weakened, fatigued, defenseless and your bodies are depleting at a more rapid pace than it's prepared for. Now your back is really vulnerable to injury from the day-to-day motions of bending, lifting, and positional changes. It all adds up, little by little, into big problems. And this is just stress and toxins we have discussed so far. Trauma is our third concern in regards to aches and pains. For the purpose of this discussion, we will define trauma as any force from outside the body that causes damage or presents injury (i.e. car accident). Remember those vertebrae, the intervertebral discs between them, and the muscles and ligaments that are supposed to bind them?

Picture now, the structure of the low back. Think about how it allows you to bend forward and backward, as well as twist to the left and to the right. Well, there are forces that affect the low back the wrong way and they are sometimes the same twisting, bending, and compression forces we were originally designed to allow. When they become traumatic, they can adversely affect your health. All you need to do is carry an object in one hand the wrong way and trip. If we then twist repeatedly in one direction or another too quickly to save the fall, the earth's gravitational forces might work against us bending backward (extension) or forward (flexion) at the waist before we fall.

Since we were lifting or carrying that object in only our one hand, we are not only tripping, but we are also falling over lopsided. The additional compression, if what you are carrying is heavy, will act on your back in an altogether worse manner.

You see, the body naturally distributes its weight evenly over the low back area of the spine. Twisting and turning, especially with weight onboard', being held by just one side of the body, causes an un-natural distribution of your weight. These forces are disastrous to the spine. Not as bad as when you'd carry a heavy weight on your shoulders or (I shiver at the thought...) on your heads, but disastrous.

In that case, the compression from the head to the neck through the mid-back down the spine to the low back and hips affects the vertebrae in a way that smashes all your discs from top to bottom. To get an idea of how this force works, picture an arrow running straight from your brain down through your spine all the way to your feet. The forces of gravity are centered in your low back (our middle) and that's where we will always feel it if we are carrying something extremely heavy or any other outside force pulls or bends us. Every time we bend over to pick up an object, and then twist one way or another...

Even to move the object while doing it, compression and grinding occurs in between the vertebrae. If any of these forces are played with repeatedly or occurs violently, the trauma inflicted could be immeasurable. Let's say you are sitting at a stoplight in your car, and another car hits you from behind. At this point, your body is violently forced to bend forward while it is thrust backward at the waist and the neck at the same time. While the lower body freezes in place, the spine is flip flopped all over the place a spring before it settles. By now, understanding a little better the structures of the back and how it moves, you can see why such an event could very easily damage your spine.

Imagine the compression forces damage to the low back spine if something falls on your head, or if you hit your head diving in a swimming pool. Shock and paralysis occurs. It is like being pinched while standing under a giant clothespin or mousetrap. Combine the pressure from above, with the ground, seemingly pushing upward, and you're suddenly crunching in the center.

You'll fold. And the damage can range from minute to extensive. Nevertheless, muscle cells, ligament fibers and intervertebral discs are torn or destroyed each and every incidence.

All this combined is what allows the spinal vertebrae to slip out of their normal alignments, secondarily impinging on the spinal nerves extending from between the vertebrae thus creating problems in all other areas of the body. Your problems can linger on for a lifetime if not taken care of properly. What if one of your traumatic experiences turns into a ruptured or herniated disc because your support structure isn't strong enough to protect itself? The discs between the vertebrae, and remember this, are made up of a tough leather-like material.

This material is arranged in several rings bound tightly together to make up the outside of the disc. In the center of the disc is a soft jelly-like substance called the nucleus propulsis. Over time if your health is neglected or your spine is damaged seriously enough, these rings can crack (rupture) and allow the soft center to move (herniate) to the outside of the disc. This can put even more direct pressure on the spinal nerves or spinal cord, causing near complete dysfunction, and compounding an already serious problem. This definitely requires treatment by a trained physician. Imagine stepping on a jelly donut. That's what I am talking about.

Every move you make, squish, squish, squish, there goes another little piece of the disc. No, not all herniated discs require surgery. In fact, 90% of them can be resolved with alternative care. In most cases, all you'll require to repair a herniated disc is moving the vertebrae back into its proper alignment. To protect ourselves, the first step is detoxification. You do that by performing enemas, getting the nutrients we need from the food we eat, the supplements we take back in order so we can restore our bodies with clean fuel to run on from day to day.

No matter what you are thinking right now, pick one of the sample diets Don has written out and stick to it despite what negative feelings you experience initially. Stick it out anyhow. Toxins leaving your body are what cause the negative feelings, like bloating, headaches, breaking out, and feeling tiresome. When 30 days have passed, you will feel wonderful! Those toxins must break free though and to do so they will have to circulate in your blood stream before they are eliminated through feces and urine. If you have a lot of them it could take a little while to eliminate. It's not that the diet isn't working, it's that you're toxic! So just stick to it - it's worth it!

Next, I want you to practice patience, relaxation and going with the flow. This will reduce stress dramatically. All things in life we call problems or issues, can either be avoided, forgotten or have pretty basic solutions. We can move past most anything with a little thought. If nothing else works, realize, there's always going to be something else popping up. So forget about it! To understand what else to do, you must first understand that what we've been talking about that happens in your spine is actually known as something called a subluxation. It is specifically defined as 'a misaligned spinal vertebra that interferes with one or more of the spinal nerves.'

Getting rid of a subluxation will get rid of most all the pain out in your body and get your health back. I have been using the term 'silent killer' because most people are sick and dying of one or more diseases such as heart disease, cancer, arthritis, tumors, and others without realizing it. They are doing things to themselves that are leading to these problems and they haven't got a clue. Diseases are all controllable, and even preventable. But a subluxation doesn't allow for healing. It leads to the subsequent deterioration of body tissues and eventually your own demise! Don't panic, I am not nuts and you aren't going to explode by morning.

Remember how I said drugs only mask the pain, but removing the cause is what helps our body to handle stress, trauma, toxins, etc? Well, removing the subluxation IS what removes the cause of the problem and therefore eliminates disease and sickness. How am I so sure? Let me explain how the body develops and functions. All people come from two cells, the sperm cell and the egg cell. The second these two cells meet in the womb they start forming more little cells and until a new life emerges. This new life is a little person made up of two parts - a physical body and a spiritual intelligence.

The spirit is what tells the physical part how to develop and function. Consequently, when a new human being starts to form, the nervous system builds itself around this spark of intelligent before anything else happens. The brain comes first, then the spinal cord, and finally, the spinal nerves grow in place. To look at it from above, the brain looks like it has a long tail attached to it, with the spinal nerves coming out in pairs from the left and right starting at the top and continuing down to the bottom. Kind of like a bean sprout, or a seed, almost.

The reason the nervous system forms first is so the intelligence, which resides inside, can send information down the spinal cord out through the nerve branches on how to form all other parts of the body. The nose, the arms, the legs, the fingers, the toes, the organs and everything else, all form normally, exactly where each belongs, based upon information coming down from the center of transmission, the brain. Eventually, this new human being (baby) develops and grows to a certain size and then it is born. The intelligence remains in the new baby and this process happens without a flinch, almost on automatic, again and again. This is why we now have a population problem. I am kidding. From this point however, it is imperative to remember that this intelligence continues to flow through the nervous system to all of the body and it's various parts to tell them how to function forever. The intelligence does this by communicating to the individual cells on a daily basis.

This system must remain constant as the human body is made up of trillions of cells and each cell or group of cells has specialized jobs to do or something is going to fail. Communication must also always be complete. For example, liver cells have a cleaning function, skin cells have a protective function, muscles have a movement function, etc.

The instruction to do all this comes from the brain, through the spinal cord, and out the spinal nerves to the cells. And it must never stop nor should it ever send the wrong message. Ever ordered a sandwich in a drive thru and the guy inside got the order wrong or you couldn't understand him? That's what happens inside of you too. The interference most typical is going to be a subluxation. Since the intelligence of the brain is supposed to be constantly sending communication, if a subluxation blocks it, you have a problem. Magnets have been used to channel this intelligence because this signal is actually an electrical current but this does not correct the subluxation.

Think of an emergency medical team shocking a person with electric pads who just had a heart attack. This intelligence inside of you is electrical, that's why they do that. When a subluxation occurs, the cells those particular nerves lead to become sick and start to die, because they lost the transmission from your brain on what to do moment by moment. But they don't all start to die right away, and that's the problem. Most of these cells live quite a while, but they live without direction. They do certain things that they are not supposed to do under these conditions and one of these things involves reproducing themselves incorrectly.

So, what you have is a group of sick cells reproducing themselves again and again somewhere in your body. You probably won't know this situation has taken place until your doctor announces you have CANCER. To understand how this happens, look at each body part and notice that the different types of cells we have replace themselves and at their own individual rates.

For example the liver replaces itself with new cells every seven months, the heart is completely renewed in five years, and the stomach lining replaces itself every four minutes. This is all vital to our existence. Cut the instruction off from the brain and our bodies have no choice but to get sick because it's already started to produce abnormal cells instead of normal ones. Sure, once in awhile we will have a symptom right away, a red light might start flashing, but this is the exception rather the rule. A subluxation occurs subtly over time, so it's over time, not over night, that we notice the multiplying group of sick cells. The symptom might be pain, numbness, tingling, or any variety of things that commonly manifest when there is a problem. This is why we need prevention.

As long as you understand that the symptom is actually the last thing to occur before you find out how bad things really are and that symptoms are only covered up and not removed by the drugs, we are on the right track. Some doctors will offer to do surgery to remove the disease too but you still won't have cut the disease off at the source this way. It always returns, because the subluxation causing it still remains, and the body will continue to create abnormal cells until you get your spine adjusted. You probably know someone who was in and out of cancer treatment for years, 'fought' so 'hard' and their doctors 'cared' so 'much' and yet they never really 'beat' it.

That's because the only doctor in the world qualified to help you with subluxations are Chiropractors. No surgery, no drugs, no amount of mumbo jumbo changes that fact. A Chiropractor first brings you in to their office and does a series of orthopedic and neurological tests including x-rays to determine where exactly the subluxation is and then they will tell you exactly how or in what way it is affecting your health. The examinations in my office also include a hands-on inspection and palpation of your spine to determine exactly where the misalignments are in the spine. Once the subluxation is then verified with the x-ray, it is corrected.

We do this through a series of painless adjustments. Depending on severity, anywhere from just one adjustment to however many more it takes to correct the problem will be scheduled one at a time. A chiropractor will not give up on you until they know you are on the right path and they will not see you any more often than necessary. Within 2 weeks of initial treatment, you will experience noticeable progress, guaranteed. From that point forward, the subluxation or misaligned vertebrae more than likely will have been removed from impinging on the nerves and then the body can truly start to heal itself naturally once again. Am I selling you something? No way.

You have already bought this book. Odds are you aren't even located anywhere near my office either. I merely want you to realize the truth behind your health. In 90% of cases reported, chiropractic care was more than helpful within 10.5 visits or 4 weeks of consistent chiropractic care than previously sought through medical care. It normally takes a series of adjustments whether we like it or not because the subluxation has probably been in the body for many years by the time we see you. When the subluxation is adjusted back into its normal alignment (from misaligned to normal alignment), it has a tendency to move back into the subluxated position at first.

This is because the body has gotten used to keeping itself in the subluxated position and must be retrained to keep the vertebrae in its most proper alignment. Through a short series of adjustments, we will retrain those muscles and ligaments that are temporarily weakened or confused. This may take time and it depends upon how long the subluxation has been there. However, unlike taking years to become ill, it doesn't take that long to begin healing again and it is also necessary to take those extra steps. It doesn't matter if you fully understand why these things are true, it matters if you know WHAT to do and that you get to work at changing your life for the better right away.

AN INTRODUCTION TO WORKING OUT

You may have attempted an exercise program before and quit. You may have found that there were time constraints and discipline requirements that were interrupted by your current lifestyle and it was just too 'difficult' to maintain everything. You may now be exercising all the time and haven't seen progress since the Berlin wall went down.

No matter what your current schedule or physical condition may be, much of what you think is a 'normal' lack of strength, flexibility, range of motion, balance, endurance, dexterity and posture, etc., all have nothing to do with aging, but rather a lack of what you do to prevent it. You probably understand that you need regular exercise, or maybe you already do, but I am also sure that you don't know what this really means. Even if you are a seasoned pro, you DON'T KNOW. Too many people are spinning their wheels, including those who are at the top of the game.

Many do not realize that the same effects of not exercising at all while we age is also what happens to us when we spend our lives exercising INCORRECTLY too. That is why many athletes are falling apart as they age. It's too much. You may want to excel at sports, tone your thighs or even build the confidence just to get out of the house and meet your soul mate. No matter the reason, you need to start the diet, not take drugs, and you need to start now, not later to get the results you want.

Exercise is the same thing you are doing when you take your car out for a drive once a week during the winter. If it just sat there for too long, the wheels would get rusty and the battery would die. Your body isn't much different. Weight lifting is the stimuli needed to start your engines, keep the wheels rolling and the key to a long lasting battery. Nutrition is the fuel of all systems involved and what the engine requires to function. Weight lifting, 'training' or 'working out' are the same things.

Each can be defined as the act of performing a various number of sets of specific repetitious movements using one or several different pieces of equipment. It is accepted that you will use a certain weight or level of resistance that is predetermined before picking up that weight as well. Simple enough. What's that really mean? Well, for example, bench presses are a single exercise and barbell curls are another. Each exercise is selected because it supposedly targets a particular muscle group.

Bench presses are selected to work your chest and barbell curls to work your biceps. Once you select an exercise, you will then determine a weight to use and probably need an idea of how many times you plan to lift it once, twice, three times or more before stopping. As far as how often to weight train, I usually suggest to my clients that they start off with a schedule where they are working out at the most every other day. It doesn't take secret equipment. Just good equipment. It doesn't take secret supplements or drugs. Just basic vitamins, minerals and essential fats along with a good diet. As far as working out 4, 5, 6 or 7 days a week... 3 days a week is sometimes too much. Even for a bodybuilder. Usually 5 workouts every two weeks with 3 of those workouts being harder than the other 2 are plenty.

So, every other session is one you will put your efforts into. I suggest putting enough effort into them that each workout shows a strength gain better than the last attempt. And no matter what, no workout should ever last more than 18 to 20 minutes in length. How much of a strength gain? I had a lady that was around 50 years old come to me back in 1997. Kathy Faix was her name. She was a nervous wreck because she was heavier than ever and had never really worked out before. She was a full time worker, married, and had two grown kids.

Those kids were in college and did I mention her cholesterol was double what it should be? Well, immediately I put her on the same program I would put anyone else on and in no time she went from 180 pounds all the way down to 140 pounds.

This might not seem good enough for people wanting to go from 140 to 120, or those looking to gain weight but bear with me. This lady lost so many inches that she began wearing clothing she hadn't worn since she weighed less than 120. She had completely restructured herself using weight training, the diet and very little aerobic exercise.

As people mature, their bones change. Keep that in mind. Your structure is always going to be a little different than it was when you were younger. But this doesn't mean you won't look better than you did when you were younger. Knowing that Kathy had a cholesterol issue and that she was passing middle age, I couldn't start her off using the weights she ended up using. We began with using a 45 pound bar for bench presses, 50 pounds on pull downs and 90 pounds (which she thought was too much).

By the end of 13 weeks, having gradually increased her resistance and diet to accommodate her building bones and strength, we not only ended up having her bench 135 pounds by herself, but doing over 600 pounds on the leg press (you read that right) and performing her own pull-ups using her bodyweight! And her cholesterol dropped hundreds of points in the process! We experienced similar results with an 80 year old retired steel worker that same year and a 30 year old client went from 160 pounds of blah to 200 pounds of athletic looking muscle doing the exact same workout Kathy used. I even had a high school kid that was considered too skinny by most standards drop 6 inches of fat off his waist and put on 35 pounds of muscle in under 9 weeks with us.

Sure, some say teenage kids exist in a naturally higher anabolic environment than what we do as adults, but that's not true. The difference isn't whether we are in our developmental years. The difference is in the amount of effort you put into your training. One thing that the older big guys do not have that the younger little guys do is the desire to push as hard as they possibly can to reach a goal. It's desire.

I think the big guys have simply lost focus after years of effort with nothing to show for it and they just do not try as hard as they used to anymore. They don't want it as much as they think they do I suppose. This high school kid however really wanted to bust out of his shell and didn't want to be the little guy on the block anymore. I also want to say that if someone is in the gym for more time than we are each session, they are foolishly doing nothing more than maintaining themselves. We trained 20 minutes at a pop, 5 sessions every 2 weeks and that's it. If you are unfamiliar with the specific exercises or machines I mention, get a complimentary training session from your gym and learn the following:

Leg Extensions, Leg Curls, and either Leg Press or Squats for your lower body. Flat Bench or Machine Chest Press and Dumbbell Flyes or Peck Deck for your chest. Overhead Military Press or Side Lateral Raises for your shoulders. Underhand Grip Pull downs and Bent Over Rows for your upper back. Tricep Pushdowns or Overhead Extensions for your triceps and either Machine or Dumbbell Curls for your biceps.

For your stomach, learn either Crunches or how to use a Nautilus Abdominal Machine that has a pad for your chest to push down upon. Trust me, learning just half these one day and the other half a second day is plenty enough to give you a 'pump.' You'll get a good workout and can switch things around for variety later on down the road. If you do desire more, I have a free web page made to show you how to perform these and several other exercises. Just email me about it if you want to practice them at home instead of wasting time wandering about clueless at a gym.

DO NOT HESITATE IN CONTACTING ME FOR THIS INFO. MOST IMPORTANT TIP OF ALL: No matter the exercise, your head must be up, your hips rotated forward, shoulder blades back, spine up right, elbows stay beside up and behind you, not on you…

And exercising less than twice a week is like not exercising at all. I do not care what Mr. Universe tells you. He was LYING. What you need to know you are about to learn. You may want to discard what you think you know before proceeding. I do not expect you to understand why this simple approach works, I merely expect you to adhere to the recommendations. I have heard, seen, tried and done it all since I began this game. I have done 2 hour long workouts, 60 minute routines and even 5 minute sessions. My best results came from reverting back to the basics almost every time, so let's begin there.

Before beginning to lift weights, you need a warm-up. You will want to move about a bit, get your juices flowing, squat down, reach over head, bend over, back, twist, turn around, jog in place for a moment. Run like Rocky up a flight of stairs if you like. Take some deep breaths and as soon as you begin to break a sweat or feel your body temperature finally matches room temperature, it's time to take your crack at the exercises. If it is really cold out you may want to warm up with a few minutes of stationary bike riding, jumping jacks or a brisk walk before weight lifting.

Only you know if that is necessary or not. I am not there to judge but always stop the warm-up once you break a sweat. Doing more than this is part of what makes you sore the next day. Believe it or not, the object is not to find out what makes you sore, but what makes you feel not so sore. Being sore isn't a sign of progress. It's a sensation caused by connective tissue damage (cumulative mirco-trauma at a cellular level) and waste that's built up from the training. Things like the amino acid hydroxy-proline becomes present after you train and it irritates your nerve endings.

You do not want this stuff trapped inside your freshly worked muscles as it hampers progress. This is the main reason why you must wait perform an aerobic (cardio) activity after you weight lift, not before. Aerobics get fresh blood into your muscles to begin the healing.

Exercise & Nutrition… The TRUTH Book One

That's really all cardio is good for until you've lost most of your fat. If you do much more than that, before you're around 10% body fat for men and 15% for women, you're going to wish you hadn't. Muscle loss anyone? Pick any one of the exercises I have mentioned or select others you know or something from the website.

One per muscle group is all you'll need and then let's begin. As either a beginner or an advanced trainer, one set per exercise is all you normally require, however, if you live in a cold environment, have low blood pressure or are nursing an injury, I am not opposed to doing a little extra something to warm up. You need mentally and physically prepared for the session. But do not waste too much energy on getting ready. Going through the motions with a lighter weight is more than enough. Sneaking something heavy in to lift masked as a warm up will only hold your progress back.

Trust me! I have NEVER met someone needing more than 3 total sets per movement and two of those were always warm ups. Ever. And that holds true only for only one or two of the exercises in the entire workout, not every exercise. The general rule of thumb is to have one warm-up for every 100 pounds of weight you plan to use. Until you can lift something heavier than your bodyweight, even doing only one set per exercise more could be too much for the time being. If you can only workout at home, either buy a compact elastic band kit or get a bench with a barbell and some extra weights. Dumbbells are a good idea, but it depends on the room you have available. I use a little of everything but for those of you on a budget, a rubber band kit really does wonders. Otherwise, with or without a barbell, squats, crunches, pushups, rear leg raises and going for a walk will work until you get that bench, barbell or rubber band kit. After the light warm-up, before you jump in and test any new exercises, I want you to next select a weight or resistance that you think allows for approximately 10 good repetitions per movement.

What is a movement? An exercise. Pick one per muscle, doesn't matter what one right now. But what exactly is a repetition? It is a single lift that consists of both a positive (or lifting) portion and a negative (or lowering) portion combined. So a rep is a one time up, and one time down motion. The amount of repetitions you perform (meaning how many times you lift a particular weight up and down again and again) per 'set' or per exercise will vary depending on your current strength, the weight you use and the goals you have. A 'set' is a collection of repetitions. If you performed 10 reps, that's a set. If you perform 2 reps, it's still a set, not a pair. A set is always going to be the complete number of repetitions you were able to perform on one exercise without stopping, doesn't matter how many that is.

I encourage you to try to do the maximum number of repetitions you possibly can each set of every exercise unless you're taking the session easy for some reason. Otherwise, I want you to work to the point of 'failure' of being able to perform another complete repetition on each set of each movement. If you do not listen to this, you will not reach your goals. And even if you can't lift the weight all the way up one more time, I want you to lower it slowly anyhow. It doesn't mean you cannot control lowering the weight even though attempts to raise it are futile.

If you have done an exercise to 'failure', and really can't perform more than you just have, the tissues have torn down to 'protect' you and prevent a continued rep. Therefore, with torn tissue, its impossible to do the same amount of reps two sets in a row. If you do 2 sets of 10, you are either not trying hard enough on the first set or you are trying much harder than you have before on the second set. Either way, it defeats the purpose. So go and attempt 15 reps next time you use a weight that allows only 10 reps on the first set. Use the same weight, try a second set, let me know if you can match those reps on the second set. If you can, you aren't listening to me. The positive or 'concentric' lifting portion of the rep may include either pulling or pushing efforts that cause the weight selected to be lifted.

Whether by cable, pulley, barbells, dumbbells or a sturdy rubber band kit, it's all the same. The raising of a weight benefits you most if you control it and take at least 4 seconds to lift. However, doing your best to control all weights so that you do not raise them faster than this is only half the battle. The other half, the negative 'eccentric' lowering motion is nothing more than the release of the weight downward towards the floor against gravity's pull.

It is considered to be the most beneficial part of the movement. This is the part of the movement that should ALWAYS be performed slowly, under as much control and released as smoothly as possible each and every repetition, especially on the very last rep you attempt to complete. 4 seconds is the fastest a rep should ever be released. That last rep should probably be released even slower. This is possible because your strength isn't in the lifting but in lowering anyhow. That's how muscle works. You'll always be able to lower more than you can lift. Lifting fights gravity, lowering works with it.

The earth is like a magnet pulling downward at your weights. Work with this magnetic effect and you will show progress in no time. We also refer to the concentric portion of the rep as either 'flexion', which is a decreasing in the angle of a joint, or the bending of a joint and 'extension' for the eccentric part which is an increasing in the angle, or the straightening of a joint. Other movements are adduction, which is the movement of a limb towards the body and abduction, which is the movement of a limb away from the body. Whatever the movement is, whatever muscle it worked, when you are done trying for more reps.... And never increase the speed on your reps just to get one more completed. That is how every single muscle injury has ever occurred... Being over zealous...

Slowly return your weight to the starting position. That is the end of your set. Now remember, I mentioned picking a weight you could lift around 10 reps with. Did you do 10? Did you not do 10?

Did you do more than 10? Write it all down. Use the KNOW HOW Log Book if you aren't sure how to keep such notes. In succeeding workouts, if you notice you have become stronger on any one exercise (being able to do more than 10 reps or even more reps than that since the previous session), you must always add a little more weight to that movement the next time you train. You do this to 'progressively' overload your ever-adapting muscles, which is what causes them to grow and your fat to burn. Letting them get used to only lifting one weight doesn't force them to work harder and that doesn't make them more efficient. So be certain to add more weight when you can handle it. If you complain of no progress, it's only because either you are not eating right or you do not try for more reps or more weight when you know darn well you should. You will keep up with this approach until your goals are met of course. After that, you can cut yourself some slack. Until then, work, work, WORK for it! So, again, if you understand what I have recommended so far, this means if you can lift a weight only 6 times, you are using too much weight.

Take some weight off or at least do not plan on adding any more weight until 10 reps are possible. If you can however lift something more than 10 times, you are not using enough weight. Add some more next time. Whether or not you are using hundreds of pounds per lift, look at this as a form of amateur bodybuilding. Listen, grandma, grandpa, you and I and any high school kid that picks up a weight is actually bodybuilding whether they like it or not. They just do not have the same goals as a professional bodybuilder. I have no interest in being big and bulky but the same rules apply to all of us. So as soon as you can lift anything for 10 repetitions without wiggling, squirming, moving your feet, lifting one side faster than the other, making faces, holding your breath, struggling much, and doing anything else otherwise considered to be cheating to lift a weight, it's time to put a few more pounds on that machine, bar, dumbbell or even add another band to the elastic kit. For now, as soon as you've finished your set, it's time to move on to another exercise.

As you go from one movement to another in subsequent sessions, you may notice that you're only getting stronger during the first half of your workout. DON'T WORRY ABOUT THIS. It is still a sign of great progress if you maintain your strength the second half. That first half should fatigue you more than before since now you are using more weight or doing more reps. So, in your higher level of fatigue, by maintaining your strength the second half of a workout, you HAVE actually gotten stronger after all.

Anytime you maintain strength when exhausted as easily as you have in the past when rested, that's progress. Also note, some muscles are just not as strong as others and do not heal within the same time frame as the bigger ones. So be patient with your body. In the months to come, that's when you can look back and determine what worked and what didn't. I say this because you also cannot always expect to show progress from one workout to another, but from one month to the next, the results will be undeniable. But realize, to stimulate the many biochemical changes within you to make this all work, training hard is necessary but it taps deep into your energy reserves. This is the key to stimulating muscle growth and fat loss, hard work.

You do need to replenish what you depleted first thing after the session. You do not grow from the actual exercises, but from what you do to allow the healing to occur through nutrition, then rest afterwards. So please consider these factors and limit each weight training session to no more than 10 different exercises and 2 sets per muscle. That's the maximum stimulation you'll ever need. I can't remember doing more than 10 sets in one workout in a long time myself. If you want more to do, or feel one exercise per muscle isn't enough variety, you should simply change your exercises and routines every now and again. I change my routine every 2 weeks but you could still make amazing progress only changing it every 30 days. Whatever you decide, immediately after training hard enough that you know you've stimulated your results, allow for them. Eat something.

What is best to start off with? If you are a beginner, I prefer you use machines (instead of barbells or dumbbells) and fight all desire to perform more than 10 sets each session including warm ups. This goes for the experienced client too. One set to failure of ten exercises is all you need to address anyone's entire body's needs in one workout. And the entire body should definitely be worked each and every session.

After that, you eat then rest a day or so. Aerobics? You do not need as much aerobic exercise working out this way. You will experience somewhat of a cardio vascular benefit by just focusing on working harder for a change. By not reserving yourself when you train, you will experience the difference your very first session. Take notice of your heavy breathing. It's undeniably aerobic. Maybe you need more of a reason than getting to do less aerobics to perform total body workouts.

Ask any physician and they will tell you that all systems of the body interrelate and none are truly independent of another. You've read what Dr. Eversole has to say about that. The body works as a whole if healthy and it's true while being trained. The chemicals stimulated, the hormones released, the work of the blood and the lungs, they all interrelate as one system with each and every exercise you do or muscle you work. It doesn't matter how you are 'splitting' up your workouts it is still stressing to the entire human system. Do you breath differently when working legs than you do working upper back or chest muscles?

You will feel the work in the area you train but you will always breath, react and recover using the same systems of the body no matter what muscles you're singling out. If you must split the workouts into halves or thirds, at least limit the amount of exercise done to no more than 30 minutes of weights or 40 minutes total, including cardio work. More advanced body builders may require more exercises, or even an extra session at times, we are talking only one or two exercises or extra sets a muscle, not 8 or 10, just ONE or TWO.

If you train incorrectly, that's one thing, but if you train too often it will nearly always result in a loss of interest for further training, having a bad attitude about your progress. You may even have headaches that occur only while exercising, possibly diarrhea will appear between sessions, yeast infections are common in over trained women, and you'll not only be exhausted all the time but anxiety and depression over your appearance will consume you to a point you'll quit... Sound familiar? They are all effects of OVER training.

'Over training' is something that happens due to the cumulative stresses your overall supporting systems experience more so than just what happened to the particular muscles you worked on a given day. The tearing down of your biceps for example with a good set of barbell curls not only affects the nerves of the bicep, but the spinal cord they are attached to and therefore the brain. At this point the body will began trying to remedy the stress of lifting that weight and tearing of muscle by getting more oxygen coming in. That's necessary in processing more nutrients and removing waste. This is why you're breathing so heavy.

And any exercise that involves a lot of heavy breathing depletes your stamina. We can agree there. For this extremely simple and scientifically valid reasoning, it makes a heck of a lot of sense that we focus on training the entire body all in one session then letting it recover before we attempt to exercise again with minimal aerobics. "If it doesn't kill you, it makes you stronger" but the body still wasn't meant to be tortured too much or tortured everyday. The added stress of over training only increases cortisol levels, which disrupts all other positive anabolic processes that you have worked so hard to enjoy. Have I scared you from exercising at all?

The next time you have a hard time catching your breath doing something as simple as climbing stairs, maybe you'll agree you need a little more activity in your life. Are you under 18 years of age? Are you over 50? Do you experience PMS?

Are you pregnant? Going bald? ALL the more reason you should begin exercising. You may need to cut the weight back a bit from what you would like to use, but you still require exercise during these important times of life more than any other.

And what we all need, even the athlete and bodybuilder, no matter how you choose to look at it, is a full body routine that tests our body's demands to stimulate results without ever over doing it. If you are a prepubescent child or anyone extremely out of shape right now who wishes to follow this exercise plan, please consult your physician and keep in touch with them until you get the hang of everything. Even though you will train on the average only 2 or 3 days a week for 20 to 30 minutes a session, it is best to have them advise you if you are currently out of shape or under 18 years of age. Getting more rest should be enough, but just in case... Talk to the doctor.

One thing is for certain, workouts this intense require more rest, so take it. This doesn't mean working out easier allows you to work out more. Easier work doesn't test you enough to do anything but maintain your appearance. We need to illicit the appropriate responses. You can potentially increase your strength by 6 times what you know it to be now following my advice but the ability to recover at most only doubles over time. What this means is you must train less often until you get stronger at first (twice a week) but once you achieve your goals, training a couple more days a week may be warranted.

Beginners can't get away with more training days for long but the experienced can train more while using heavier weights. I consider that a luxury. I can go to the gym and train, run a mile and be completely done with everything in 30 minutes 2 or 3 days a week because I am no longer looking to set personal strength records. Nothing beats that! If you are able to bench, squat, and barbell row your own weight for 10 reps minimum each, you can add an extra workout to the schedule.

If not, 3 sessions a week are plenty. If you are thinking right now that aerobics must be an easier way to get started, it isn't. Even if you are reduced to lifting feathers at first, or must cut the weight you use back to what you used as a teenager in order to perform each movement correctly, weight training is still the single most beneficial form of exercise in regards to reaching all our goals. Can you ever workout out more often than 3 times one week and 2 times the next? If you like, sure, but if you aren't progressing by getting fitter or stronger each and every session, what do you really think you'll need next? More workouts or more rest? Remain patient with me here. If you work hard enough on at least working at increasing your weaknesses each session, but not so hard you blow a piston, even only short term, and you will get the results you seek.

Forget about entering a physique contest or becoming the Incredible Hulk right now. If that's the plan, it will happen in time. For now, focus only on your weaknesses twice a week. Do this and your weaknesses will vanish within no time and you won't worry about 3 sessions a week. I bet you're also curious why I recommend only doing enough movement to break a small sweat before training. How can that be enough of a warm up to prevent injury?

When you select a weight that you think you can perform no more than 10 repetitions with under slow and controlled movement (remember, you're taking 4 seconds to raise the weight and 4 seconds to lower it without yanking or dropping it), by the time those ten reps are complete, a good 80 seconds should have passed. It only takes 30 seconds to properly warm a joint up. How so? If you take your time and lift a weight 4 seconds up, control lowering it down for another 4 seconds, that's 8 seconds a complete rep. After 4 reps, or 32 seconds later, enough blood has been squeezed from your working muscles into your cold and stiff tendons to 'warm' and 'loosen' them up.

This is the most natural process in protecting your ligaments and tendons. By the time the 10th rep comes around, you are probably as safe as anyone could ever hope to be as long as you aren't getting sloppy with your form. Cold tendons are like plastic, warm tendons are like rubber. If you move slow and always get the form correct before deciding to add weight to an exercise, you'll never need a formal warm up or have the pleasure of experiencing an injury. I have, and I know first hand that injuries only occur from sudden jerks like catching a refrigerator falling off a truck to save your child (Lou Ferrigno did this once).

So do not throw your weights around and you will be fine. This is why I also say it's important to get the art of movement down first or have the opinion of someone watching you, like a trainer, or a workout partner at all times. A 'spotter' is someone who guides you through the 'spots' you have trouble. You don't need to invest a lot of money in a trainer if you need one at first. The commitment is to yourself and not to the trainer. In fact, make it clear to them you are going to try one or more trainers for a session or two each so you can learn what you can about basic movements, then you plan to move on. If you doubt any one of them in any way, do not train with them any longer.

Maybe you can think of someone at work who you can ask to show you a few of the exercises mentioned in this book. Maybe you live with such a person that can help. Maybe you are related to someone who can offer guidance. If not, this is no excuse to give up. Start now by calling the gym for a one time trainer referral or look through the yellow pages. Call just one person and request just one session. Tell them you do not want a workout, you simply want them to teach you a few exercises.

From there, you will be able to build a foundation on your own. Sound simple enough? It is but it's something you requires 100% of your dedication. If you want results, I want you to clear your head of all things when you begin a movement.

Concentrate on nothing else around you. The only thing that should matter while in the gym is the exercise. Block everything else out. It is essential to be in tune with your body and the motions it performs. You want to become 'one' with the task at hand and 'center' your mind along with your very existence in the experience of lifting a weight. For instance, when I work on a bicep machine, I focus on listening to my breathing from the inside and out.

I feel my biceps pulling the weight upwards while it contracts to lift and then I enjoy the feel of the handles slowly stretching the muscles as it pulls back down again lowering the weight. I pay close attention not to extend too far down or pull up too fast either. I reverse the downward movement at the exact same point each and every time to bring the weight back again too. I am aware throughout the set that my grip is not tight but relaxed. The handles or bar simply rests in the palm of my hands and is cradled as I control it. My hands are merely hooks as I feel the bicep do all my work.

I know how far up to raise the weight and I know that no one is too close to bump the bar. I see all around me without looking. I keep my head straight and I breath in and out without thought. I am not looking away from the floor for anything as I continue to focus on each repetition until I am sure one more is absolutely impossible. I never hold my breath while lifting even as the work gets harder. I keep my air passages open during all phases of the exercise to supply my body with enough oxygen to get me through the work it is doing. Holding your breath can elevate your blood pressure to dangerously high levels and contribute to a self-induced headache. If you do begin to experience a headache while training, even a mild one, slowly return to the starting position and stop the exercise immediately. Start taking in deep breaths and develop a rhythmic pattern like you are jogging to stick with throughout each movement. Breath in and breath out several times a rep if necessary. NEVER hold it.

I try for more and more reps AGAIN AND AGAIN without flinching until I can no longer do so. The objective to training is to work harder than you did last time. That means when discomfort arises, like burning inside the muscle, ignore it. The feeling is temporary. Never stop midway. I will continue to raise the weight in 4 seconds, pause at the top barely a second just to be sure I feel the muscles are contracted, then I will lower the weight just as slowly as I raised it. If the weight seems heavier as I do more and more reps it might take 5 seconds or more to raise in those later reps. If this happens, take 5 seconds to lower it too.

It may take 6 or 7 seconds to raise and lower the weight. Once you get to the last rep, I know I must try for a full five more seconds to move the weight anyhow. Even if it only raises a hair more, I do not stop until I know for sure the weight just isn't going to budge. When I am certain the weight is not capable of being raised any further, I slowly lower the bar (which you are always capable of doing because remember, the lowering portion of a rep is where the muscle remains the strongest) and then put it back into the starting position. I stop for just a moment afterward to take a deep breath into the bottom of my lungs then get up to prepare for the next exercise. I might stretch the muscle I just worked, or I might not. But I waste no time getting to my next movement.

Slow movers have slow metabolisms. I do not rush THROUGH a set. I rush TO the set. I realize when some sets are complete, allowing for 'just' enough time to go on to the next movement may seem impossible. Not just because you must wait for someone else to get off a machine, but because working hard and trying for ten reps with something you can barely do 9 with is grueling. I have been winded for up to 15 minutes after a hard leg press or squat, but I don't stop. I move on. If you rest much longer than two minutes, you lose your anabolic edge (muscle building and fat burning potential) and your joints will 'cool' down. We don't want that to happen.

This is also why your workouts are limited to 10 sets and 10 to 12 minutes of total aerobics. No total workout should last more than 40 minutes or you're defeating the purpose of being there. You lose the hormonal boost you get from training if you 'lolly gag' around. The minute that it takes you to walk from one machine to the next is quite enough time to get mentally ready for more work. For the best results, it is important to feel completely rested and vigorous at the beginning of every workout, not necessarily between sets. Sorry, but I do not expect you to enjoy the work. I expect you to enjoy the RESULTS.

What sort of aerobics AKA...cardio work? Again, riding a bike, a rowing machine, climb a stair master, take a jog or paddle an aerodyne if you like as they all will suffice. Whichever you select, hop on your machine of choice and perform 12 nonstop minutes of serious huff and puff and don't hold back. Write down how far you travel during the exercise (150 flights of stairs, 3.5 miles, 10 kilometers, etc) and at what speed you traveled at (4 MPH of KPH, etc) in your Know How Log. If you want results, I recommend trying as hard as you can for at least 10 and no more than 15 minutes each session.

Try to achieve more distance in the same amount of time worked as often as you possibly can. I realize an average of 12 minutes doesn't seem like much but it truly is plenty for now. The reason being is that despite most people believing that after 20 minutes of cardio work your body begins fat burning, it's only true if the body has burnt it's glycogen the first 20 minutes you trained. The problem here is that the body burns a lot of amino acids (muscle) along with its glycogen during the initial 20 minutes of endurance movement. And if you keep going at it for more than 40 minutes, you'll burn even more muscle.

So while you have a 20 minute 'window of opportunity', so to speak, in the middle for fat burning after the glycogen is burned, doesn't it make sense to do something which doesn't burn muscle so all you burn is fat? That would be weight lifting!

If you lift weights first you'll deplete of glycogen, preserve muscle, then when you exercise from the 20 to 40 minute time frame, you'll burn nothing but fat. However, let's assume if you're not at 10% body fat for men or 15% body fat for women yet, your body is normally 'storing' more fat than it burns.

If this is true, then your body's preferred energy sources are more than likely muscle tissues. This is why you aren't as tone as you want to be and when your fat levels are low, your muscles are fuller looking. If you grasp this concept, then you'll understand that when I say aerobics really only burn whatever your body's current preferred energy sources are for fuel, you won't want to do too much cardio work right now. If you're still fat, then those first 40 minutes of exercise (20 or 30 minutes with weights and 10 to 15 minutes of cardio) are plenty for now. Let your diet peel the fat away. Otherwise, more cardio only means you're going to stay fat. Why would you want to argue this matter? I am trying to save you time!

I do something on occasion I call HIGH intensity aerobics where I run hard as nails for 10 minutes, then I reduce my speed to 80% of that intensity for another 5 minutes. I reserve this sort of aerobics for ONLY AFTER a weight session. Occasionally upon waking, performing aerobics is good too but only if you are already able to see your abdominal muscles, but do not start such a schedule before that. And 3 days a week of 20 minutes in the morning adds up to an hour a week MAX, not an hour per session, an hour extra per week too. You will NEVER break a sweat as quickly as when doing this sort of high intensity aerobics. Another version I made popular back in 1992 that a well known magazine ripped off from me just a few years back was where I would run for 3 minutes hard, then one minute slow, followed by 3 minutes hard, and one minute slow again for 3 complete cycles... It's AWESOME if you will do it right. Problem is, again, not many people CAN run for 3 minutes all out then only take a minute to jog at a slower pace and still be able to run another 3 minutes as fast as possible one more time.

What happens is that they jog for 3 minutes then walk, then jog and that's not the point. If this is you, try the same routine on a stationary bike or rowing machine. See how it works. Finding what fits your interest is what keeps you coming back for more each session. I use another high intensity approach to aerobic training too. The workout begins by riding my bike at a steady pace for a minute, then I increase the intensity to a higher level that has me crying to myself to quit for a full three minutes and then I go back to the easier level for a minute. Next, you guessed it, another three minutes of hard core cycling followed by one minute to cool down a little at a slower pace. Then you do this one more time and you are done.

Sounds simple but try riding at a high enough level that you'll want to quit after 15 seconds but knowing you aren't allowed to, just keep going and HATE IT but DO IT. Another cardio regime I perform involves pedaling on a bike at the lowest level for 30 seconds, which is usually Level One and increasing the levels one at a time each additional 30 second increment. Most machines go up to 12 Levels. So in six minutes, when I am at the highest level and am halfway through the 12 minute session, I decrease one notch at a time just as I increased them. I pedal my bike as hard as my body allows until my time is up and I am back at level one again.

If you cannot make it to the top level, that is alright. Divide the time left by however many levels you completed to finish your session. If you made it to level 4 in 2 to 4 minutes, divide the remaining 8 to 10 minutes by 4, which is 2 and a half or 2 minutes and 30 seconds before you decrease the levels again. You will get it in time. Guess what. If you weight train like I suggest, you can do ANYTHING you want aerobically for these 12 minutes and you will burn fat anyhow. I look at these twelve minutes as important because they force your blood vessels to create new route openings for delivering fresh oxygen to nourish your muscle tissues.

Without this, you do not heal properly. This is what is meant by "Max VO2 uptake". It is the efficiency that oxygen is taken to the cells with nutrients to heal you. Realize, most of your life (90%) is spent performing anaerobic muscular generated movements, not aerobics. If you want to look like those fat ladies on the aerobics machines who ride, stair climb and treadmill themselves into the ground 2 hours a night and who after months still don't look any better, then sit this book down or give it away. You're not ready for the truth. Otherwise, the closer you pay attention to me, and the harder you work... The more progress you will make. After cardio, that's when you should do some stretches, but nothing else and do not take forever about it. If I did not stretch between sets, where I normally have my partner or my 'assistant' stretch me, you can bet I did them after my workout. If I am alone, that's no excuse, I still do them by myself. I DO NOT stretch as a warm up. That's looking for trouble. Your tendons are brittle when cold. Stretch only after you've worked. It'll feel so good as the sensation of fresh blood flushes into your newly worked muscles.

In case you, your trainer or your partner do not understand stretching techniques, you may want to watch one of my video cassettes that demonstrate these procedures. After your workout, our bodies need carbohydrate foods and liquids. I suggest you have a half sized carb meal directly after the routine and a regular full sized protein meal 90 minutes following that. Not eating protein with a little fat (whey protein and cream is my choice) before a workout or having carbs afterwards then more protein 90 minutes again later will cause your body to cannibalize it's own muscle tissue. It does this looking for either recovery nutrients or the energy it needs to rebuild, otherwise defeating the purpose of the working out to begin with. You should eat well all the time and drink plenty of water before, during AND after your workouts. But most of you are already willing to do this much. Just don't fall into the trap of having carbs before or during a workout (THAT'S REAL BAD) and waiting to eat them after. This is not good.

Carbs during a session lead to dehydration, which reduces your blood volume and missing them afterwards causes you to store rather than burn fat too. So DRINK ONLY WATER and plenty of it to wash down those post workout carbs.

No matter what, you should also try to rest your body by not training at all (including aerobics) at least 48 hours between every single workout (light activity is fine on your 'off' days, but no weights are to be lifted and no tough aerobic sessions). Many people like to alternate between weights on one day and cardio-vascular exercise on the next. I would recommend against this. Rest and rest WELL. You will succeed faster. It is the resting periods between workouts that the body builds muscle and burns fat. Without sufficient rest, you make no progress.

You see, growth and fat loss do not take place until after the muscles have fully recuperated. Exercise damages you. The body requires recuperation or 'recovery' time after each session. It's healing. Like with a scab. You pick, you pick, and you bleed some more. Just let the wound heal. An EMS unit or getting a massage between sessions to speed healing is helpful but not crucial. No EMS machine is helpful in giving you amazing abs though...

Please note: When you are not at home and on the road traveling, it's all right to take an extra day off between sessions if that is what your schedule is calling for. Just make sure you get 2 sessions in a week. If you do not think you have time to get to a gym, try to make the time. Nobody, no matter how successful or busy they think they are should avoid taking a half hour to devote to a training session at least twice a week. Find a gym, get yourself to it, knock the workout off and feel good about it. Put yourself first at least twice a week. If this is impossible, then schedule a session for right before leaving town and another upon returning home. Either that or get yourself a good elastics band kit. But workout one way or another. You need it.

While we are all individuals and different, we are still all so much the same that we do not require that much more or less than the next person does, so the rules that apply to you apply to virtually anyone. In advanced cases we may take things like specific workout frequency, intensity, time, reps, environment and the type of exercise you are doing into consideration but to produce desired results, a bench press is a bench press and a row is a row and a squat is a squat.

Older folk always heal more slowly. Not that 40 is old, but physical changes manifest after age 30 that tend to slow our healing a bit. If you are over 40, you better take heed. Learn to read your body. Focus. Feel each heart beat when you breath. Feel each movement you perform. Know what you are doing. Feel the stretch and contraction as you lift and lower the weights.

Come to understand any and all feedback from your body. Take notes and come to be able to instantaneously interpret feedback appropriately in order to achieve continued results. This is why you came to me. Sometimes we need to call in a driver when the road gets rough. Not that weight training is like brain surgery, but unless you create automatic habits out of these things, it's going to feel like pulling teeth just to lose or gain a pound. Like you have created bad habits over time, these are the good ones I want you to adopt today. And do not be afraid to ask for a trainer's advice if necessary.

But if their advice extends further than how to perform the exercises I recommended or differs from what you have read in this chapter so far, smile, say 'thanks anyhow' and walk away. The only thing you need to learn from anyone else now is, possibly, where a particular machine is located in the gym. The rest is within these pages. No matter your level of fitness, the only difference between most of you and the trainers you speak to anyhow is the amount of weight you use when you train.

THE FOUR PHASES OF WEIGHT TRAINING

For years, I have told people that if they are not getting stronger they merely need a little more time between workouts to rest their muscles. Recovery, growth and fat loss all occur out of the gym. Not in it. Weight lifting is simply the stimuli needed to produce your results and getting a pump, sweaty or sore means nothing in the way of progress. Disagree?

Go tonight to the gym or whatever day you workout next and then cancel all days off for a while. That's right, I want you to go to the gym every single day but only until a session proves to be fruitless. That means I want you to go every single day until you see a noticeable decline in your strength. Eventually you will encounter the inability to improve, maybe you already have, but do this anyhow. And keep notes.

Unfortunately, you aren't going to get anywhere regardless of your commitment without knowing what the heck you're doing wrong first so do this for me. Once your strength noticeably decreases, that's when I want you to take a day off. Go every other day from that point forward and if you can't add weight or do more reps at one of the subsequent workouts, add an extra day of rest between each session until you can. It will makes sense soon enough.

I do want these workouts to be total body workouts by the way. No 2 way, 3 way, 4 way or whatever way splits you are accustomed to. Perform one exercise per muscle group and select only a weight you know you can handle for around 12 reps. Even if you are currently lifting feathers for 12 reps, you can expect to see dramatic strength increases as each month passes if you follow this rationale. Results come from recovery and you cannot expect to recover unless you rest. You will see after you come back with just that first day off without exercising at all. Tell me then whether your strength went up or not. I bet it does.

If not, take another day off until your next session. I am certain you will be stronger that time. The key is finding a groove of how much effort versus how much rest you require as an individual. And when you get into that groove, pay attention to your patterns and you will know when you need either one, two or maybe three days off between sessions to assure progress.

Who could possibly know this sort of information for either you or a client until you or they at least tested yourselves accordingly? You couldn't. Since I want you to take me up on the training every day until progress halts challenge, here is how we manipulated it for prime results with one of my own former clients. I will also explain how and where to break things down into its four different phases.

Phase One.

Work out every day using a full body workout just to get the kinks out of the new routine and your muscles. Use this time to learn the movements, figure out what you're supposed to feel and make sure your joints are feeling right. When you train with weights, which you must, you break down muscle and it fills up with waste that makes you sore.

Working out every day at first keeps the waste flushing out of your muscles until the body starts doing it more efficiently on it's own. Even if you are more experienced that the next person, I would still try out my new routine every day for a spell until my strength goes down too. This isn't a test for just beginners.

It's something I do with all of my clients because I also know if I told them to start off with just 2 sessions a week, they wouldn't listen to me nor believe such a thing could work. So, for the time being, go workout every single day until you start to lose strength. It might halt on you after your second, third or tenth session, nobody knows just yet.

Wherever it does stop, that's when and only when you will begin taking a day of rest off between sessions. In your training log you should list what exercises you have done, the weights used, the reps performed and I will show you how in a moment. Also note the dates and everything else, which the Know How Log (see www.RefuseToFail.com) asks for after or during each individual session. Here is how our first three sessions might go as they did with my one client.

"WO" is short for workout, so "WO1" for instance means "workout number one" and 185 x 12 means we used 185 pounds for 12 repetitions... The exercise is listed and followed by the first three session results. Also note, the rules apply to both men and women. If a lady wants to lose fat, she must work for it. Muscles will not appear on you overnight like it seems with men. I promise.

Squat - WO1: 185 x 12, WO2: 185 x 15, WO3: 185 x 13
Bench - WO1: 185 x 8, WO2: 185 x 10, WO3: 185 x 9
Bent Over Row - WO1: 145 x 6, WO2: 145 x 8, WO3: 145 x 8
Pull Downs - WO1: 140 x 6, WO2: 140 x 8, WO3: 140 x 8
Military Press - WO1: 100 x 10, WO2: 100 x 12, WO3: 105 x 10
Leg Extension - WO1: 90 x 12, WO2: 100 x 12, WO3: 110 x 10
Leg Curls - WO1: 70 x 14, WO2: 80 x 15, WO3: 80 x 14
Machine Curls - WO1: 70 x 8, WO2: 70 x 10, WO3: 80 x 10
Lat Pushdowns - WO1: 70 x 13, WO2: 80 x 13, WO3: 80 x 10

Notice how our client got stronger from one workout to the next and then all of a sudden lost strength? This could take 2 sessions or 20 sessions. We are all different. Keep going until you lose strength too. Keep in mind that while this client IS a real person, and these are his REAL results, you are individual and should not use these exercises unless you are familiar with them nor these weights unless you are capable of lifting them.

The idea is to use a weight for as many reps as you can too, not to stop at a set figure because you see it here. Test yourself....

And do not try to follow this plan by training only on the same days he did either. It may benefit you, but it won't be optimal as these aren't your results.

Note that sometimes your strength may only drop on a few exercises, maybe all of them or even just one. However, even if just one set on one lone exercise falls short of making progress, it is time to continue and finish the session, keep notes, go home, rest, eat, sleep and do not return for two days.

Remember though, if you could do 10 or 12 reps the last session you should have added weight the next time. This will most always inadvertently decrease the amount of reps you do because it is heavier weight you are using, but that's the idea. To make the exercise harder to perform again.

Either way, after that first day off you will be stronger again on virtually everything and that is evidence that recovery requires an occasional break. Another reason to rest is to develop your joints, tendons, and ligaments too. They all heal very slowly in comparison to a muscle. You see, a joint is where two bones meet. A tendon is what attaches muscle to bone and then ligament attaches bone to bone.

Phase Two.

This is when you begin to work out every other day. Picking up your next session after a complete day of rest, look at your notes and see if you got stronger or not. If you did, great, rest one more day again and then add weight to the exercises you saw the most results with the next session. If you add 5% more weight, understand that the reps should drop by 10% because it is tough sometimes to tolerate the additional pounds and continue to do the same amount of reps as before. It's heavier after all. Think about it. Here were our phase two results after training every other day until progress became inconsistent...

Squat - WO1: 185 x 16, WO2: 195 x 15, WO3: 205 x 13
Bench - WO1: 185 x 12, WO2: 195 x 10, WO3: 205 x 9
Bent Over Rows - WO1: 145 x 10, WO2: 145 x 12, WO3: 165 x 8
Pull Downs - WO1: 140 x 9, WO2: 140 x 12, WO3: 160 x 8
Military Press - WO1: 105 x 12, WO2: 110 x12, WO3: 115 x10
Leg Extension - WO1: 110 x12, WO2: 110 x 15, WO3: 120 x 10
Leg Curls - WO1: 80 x 18, WO2: 90 x 15, WO3: 100 x10
Machine Curls - WO1: 80 x 12, WO2: 90 x 12, WO3: 100 x 10
Lat Pushdowns - WO1: 80 x 15, WO2: 90 x 13, WO3: 100 x 8

In just 6 days of training (3 sessions 'on' and 3 days 'off') his progress came really quick and also allowed for considerable increases in weight. We went on like this (training every other day) for another week before his strength declined.

It was exciting for both of us. In under 3 weeks, he was stronger than he had ever been in his life. And at that point I suggested we start training every third day. We did finish that one last workout but after that we took two days off before returning again…

Phase Three.

Sooner or later, like it or not, even working out just once every other day will be too much for the body to handle. But hey, if it means continued results, who cares how often you train? As long as it works, right? So if there comes a day you just do not feel like working out, even though you were stronger the last time you trained, like maybe you feel your strength isn't there, then it's time for the next phase.

If you feel really good, ready to go, exploding with energy, that's the difference between progressing and over training. With this particular client, after a phase of every other day training and great progress, then taking two days off, the results just kept coming.

We added 2 or 3 reps to each exercise and even had him handling more weight on several movements week after week too. And he was looking GREAT. However, due to the incredible strength gains and maintaining the old rule of thumb (working the heavier exercises first and working down to the lightest weights last), we rearranged the exercises a little.

Squat - WO1: 235 x 16, WO2: 245 x 15, WO3: 255 x13
Bench - WO1: 215 x 12, WO2: 225 x 10, WO3: 225 x 8
Bent Over Row - WO1: 185 x 10, WO2: 185 x 12, WO3: 195 x 6
Pull Downs - WO1: 180 x 9, WO2: 180 x 12, WO3: 190 x 8
Leg Extension - WO1: 150 x 12, WO2: 160 x 15, WO3: 170 x 10
Military Press - WO1: 125 x 12, WO2: 130 x 12, WO3: 135 x 6
Leg Curls - WO1: 120 x 18, WO2: 130 x 15, WO3: 140 x 10
Lat Pushdowns - WO1: 120 x 15, WO2: 130 x 13, WO3: 140 x 8
Machine Curls - WO1: 110 x 12, WO2: 120 x 12, WO3: 130 x 10

We went a fourth session after that and the reps went up even further but during that final session, everything slipped. The next phase called for 3 days off between sessions…

Phase Four. This is the final phase before beginning an entirely brand new workout routine. Three of the exercises were rearranged again to move the heavier movements up the list and the lighter ones closer to the bottom. The only time you would work smaller or weaker muscles first is if you are trying to pick up parts of you that are out of proportion.

I sometimes do legs last in my session, just before I perform cardio but this depends on my current routine. With this particular client, after performing sessions between 3 days of rest, Phase Four eventually required just two sessions a week to see continued results.

Squat - WO1: 275 x 12, WO2: 285 x 12, WO3: 295 x 13
Bench - WO1: 235 x 10, WO2: 225 x 12, WO3: 230 x 8
Pull Downs - WO1: 210 x 8, WO2: 210 x 12, WO3: 220 x 8

Bent Over Row - WO1: 205 x 8, WO2: 205 x 12, WO3: 215 x 9
Leg Extension - WO1: 190 x 10, WO2: 190 x 15, WO3: 200 x 10
Leg Curls - WO1: 160 x 10, WO2: 160 x 13, WO3: 170 x 10
Military Press - WO1: 150 x 10, WO2: 150 x 12, WO3: 155 x 7
Lat Pushdowns - WO1: 150 x 10, WO2: 150 x 13, WO3: 160 x 8
Machine Curls - WO1: 140 x 10, WO2: 140 x 12, WO3: 150 x 10

We progressed marvelously for 5 more sessions at just twice a week after that. Things came to an end at around nine weeks (remember, this is just an example of one client, sometimes all four phases are exhausted in more or less time than that, I have seen it last only a month and up to 4 months). Looking back, we performed just 23 sessions over a mere 9 weeks, which produced the following results from workout one to workout twenty three...

Squat WO1: 185 x 12, After 63 Days... WO23: 335 x 13
Bench WO1: 185 x 8, After 63 Days... WO23: 260 x 8
Pull Downs WO1: 140 x 6, After 63 Days... WO23: 250 x 8
Bent Over Row WO1: 145 x 6, After 63 Days... WO23: 235 x 9
Leg Extension WO1: 90 x 12, After 63 Days... WO23: 250 x 10
Leg Curls WO1: 70 x 14, After 63 Days... WO23: 200 x 10
Military Press WO1: 100 x 10, After 63 Days... WO23: 175 x 7
Lat Pushdowns WO1: 70 x 13, After 63 Days... WO23: 180 x 8
Machine Curls WO1: 70 x 8, After 63 Days... WO23: 160 x 10

How did he get so strong? Four reasons. One. He wasn't trying hard enough on these exercises when I first met him. He needed a little motivation. Once he had it, which all good trainers provide, he put more effort into things. Two. He wasn't eating enough food when we met.

At first I had to force feed him to some extent but as we progressed, he just couldn't eat enough! He went from 2000 calories a day to 5000 calories a day by adding around 300 calories a week. Women may only add 50 calories a week, but that too is necessary to burn body fat.

I know you think that by exercising a lot you can get away with not eating right, but it will catch up. You may trick the body into maintaining muscle for a while but it cannot build any extra if the diet doesn't supply the concrete for your foundation. If you would just stop working out so often, let the body heal, change the eating habits, the body would not only look more tone but drop a heck of a lot of fat. Three. Like I said, he wasn't resting between sessions before he met me. He was training every day and then after a while, he would burn out and give up then not train at all for months on end. There was no consistency to his routine.

Four. He gained 40 pounds! That is correct, 40 pounds. He went from 150 to 190 in 63 days. Now, I know what you are thinking ladies. This isn't going to happen to you. Women do not possess enough testosterone to bulk up so fast.

Here is the calendar for those two months I trained our mystery client:

Sun Mon Tues Wed Thurs Fri Sat

Week 1 rest WO WO WO rest WO rest
Week 2 WO rest WO rest WO rest WO
Week 3 rest WO rest WO rest rest WO
Week 4 rest rest WO rest rest WO rest
Week 5 rest WO rest rest WO rest rest
Week 6 rest WO rest rest WO rest rest
Week 7 rest WO rest rest WO rest rest
Week 8 rest WO rest rest WO rest rest
Week 9 rest WO rest rest WO rest rest

I have seen success with training 5 days straight, taking a day off, training 4 days straight, taking a day off, training 3 days straight, taking a day off, training 2 days straight, taking a day, training one day on and one day off after that and expanding to 2 days off when necessary. I think you get the picture.

PHASE FIVE?

After phase four, you should come up with an all new workout plan using all new exercises (thus maintaining variety) and start all over again at phase one or start the 3 days one week and 2 days the next routines I have mentioned so often before. You could also work out 3 days a week every week, making the middle session an easy workout. You could also take what you have discovered and draw up a schedule of your own.

It's up to you. No matter what you do, the results will never duplicate, but they will keep coming if you apply the resting principles. It is safe to assume you could follow this type of schedule for at least a year. I don't see any reason why you couldn't go on forever using the Four Phases actually. I however split my year up, periodizing it as they say, into cycles. A 'micro' cycle would be a specific workout.

A 'meso' cycle would be the 1, 2, 3 or 4 months I am training for a specific goal like using the same weights for a certain period and simply trying to get more and more reps as time goes on or increasing my strength instead.

And finally a 'macro' cycle could be the entire year or a 6 month period of macro cycles combined together working towards meeting another specific goal. I suggest spending 3 months a year maintaining your physique, 3 months working on weak points, 3 months trying to drop any fat gained during the holiday season so you look good at the beach and 3 months experimenting with whatever routines you enjoyed in the past or have wanted to try for a while. In fact, you do not need to change exercises at all if you do not feel like it. I spent a whole year doing just leg presses, seated machine rows, and seated chest presses once. If I felt up to it, I added a few other exercises, sure, but no matter what, I regularly performed just these three main exercises and made GREAT progress that year too.

If my strength slipped, I took my days off but I also wouldn't perform the extra movements until my strength went back up again. This worked because I periodized the intensity cycles of what my goals were month to month. My goals that year were divided into periods of lower intensity work and periods of high intensity training. These periods should be based on your "One Rep Max." What is that? There is no getting around the fact that exercise is a science, but in order for a muscle to develop, there is a simplicity to this that definitely differs it from rocket science.

All a muscle needs for development is trained regularly with a resistance greater than the outside forces it is accustomed to encountering and in a variety of intensities if possible. While training for a few months straight, even if you make promising results, you will eventually grow tired or over trained no matter how close you pay attention to your progress.

You can keep adding weight every time you are capable of performing 10 or more reps on any particular movement, or even take days off when you need it, but something will be missing and something will end up stalling. That is unless you also use the precise repetition range that each of our individual muscle groups require.

As with everything else, not only are there certain exercises, but perceived intensity differentials per muscle group that must be taken into consideration. Athlete or not, our muscles were designed each for different uses and one rep range isn't going to cover the needs (nor development) for all of them very long.

Your 'one rep max' (1RM) is the maximum amount of weight you can do using a certain weight on a certain exercise that you can barely muster for one repetition with and momentarily will not have the strength to perform a second rep with, no matter how hard you try. You will of course not attempt to determine your one rep max as a beginner and it's probably not even necessary at intermediate levels.

It is a tool used by clients who are more advanced to find what 80% of their one rep maximums per each muscle group are. Once you know that info you can reach new heights in your training. For instance, say you can bench 150 pounds for one rep but not two. That's your one rep max, 150 pounds. 80% of 150 is 120 so 120 pounds is your 80% max. Follow me so far?

While you already know that each muscle group maintains a different level of strength, each muscle also will own a different rep range while using 80% of it's one rep max weight. The difference in the reps performed using 80% of your one rep max is the gauge of the difference in recovery ability from not only individual to individual but muscle to muscle. That's what makes this info so important to seasoned clientele.

What I mean is, by controlling your rep ranges, your individual muscles will not need more or less time to recover than the others and you can actually almost know for certain when or when not to train too. This method works because it determines what type of predominant fiber you have in each muscle.

Instead of worrying about your 80% ranges and one rep maxes, or rotating intensity levels workout to workout, unless you're an advanced client, for now, if you do sets to failure with 30, 8 and 12 reps, you will address all your different muscle fiber type needs. Your best bet in this case if you ask me is to train 3 days a week.

Monday perform 8 reps each exercise (or close to it), Wednesday perform 30 reps and on Fridays 12 reps. But because we have different muscle fiber types in each muscle and while 80% does in fact work the largest percentage of them, which is what stimulates both fat loss and muscle building, that's what I want to focus on for the time being.

However, the fibers are completely different. One type of muscle fiber is a red. It is a slow twitching, smaller type and somewhat aerobic fiber. The second is an intermediate, somewhat fast twitching, medium sized, mostly aerobic type fiber. And the third group, the white, fast, large, and anaerobic type fiber is usually most predominant and what we seek to work by using 80% of our one rep max weights.

There is a fourth, which is basically the same type as the third, and it to is recruited by using the heavier weights or 80% ranges. To work the other fibers I simply double my reps once and then double them again by changing the weights I use for different points in my periodization program.

Say per muscle, using the 80% range as a goal, you can perform 4 reps on thigh exercises, then to work muscle fiber group number two, try doubling the reps performed by lowering the weight used (in this case you would be doing sets of 8 reps instead of 4). To better work the first group of red muscle fibers, you would lower the weight even more and double the reps again (going from 8 reps to 16). I do not know if 4 is the number of reps you are working with, that's something you will need to discover.

It's just an example. Maybe your hamstrings allow for 10 reps with 80% of your one rep max. I would then also perform 20 and 30 rep sets somewhere in my schedule to make sure the muscles are fully developed.

Another thing, even if you are able to bench, squat, and barbell row your own weight for 10 reps minimum each, you ARE STILL NOT ready to test for a one rep max. When you can bench, row and squat 50% more than you weigh, I am still not convinced you should bother. But if you are truly wanting to look like a bodybuilder or become an athlete, you might want to do this. How so?

You find your one rep max by having your partner help you to find what is the heaviest weight you can use for only one rep on one exercise for each of your different muscle groups.

Any exercise for any muscle could be selected. It may take you a few sets to figure out, a few tries, who knows, but be sure the weight you come up with only allows for 1 rep not 2 and do not try on so many sets that you aren't absolutely certain of the results. If you pick the weight up and it feels like you can do more than one, STOP. Add more weight.

Once you are there with the right weight, do one rep then try one and take a break. Three minutes is plenty enough time. Afterwards, perform one more set using 80% of that weight. Write down the results then rest two days. Next, go back and do just one set with the same 80% poundages again. You should notice that you are a few reps stronger on each exercise.

Make sure you write this down so you know how much stronger. Compare the figures from day one to the new ones. Day one you may have mustered 6 reps but on day two you probably got 8. Maybe it was 12 to 15. Only you can determine this but whatever it is, this is now your rep range for each exercise. If you are doing this with a friend or a client you will now see that 80% ranges of a one rep max results really do vary from person to person and muscle to muscle.

As time passes by using these %'s in your workouts, I want you to add weight to whatever movement you need to whenever you can do more than your higher-end rep ranges, but not so much you fall below your lower-end ranges. If your rep range is supposed to stay with in 8 to 10 reps for a particular muscle in order to garnish the greatest results, and you can perform 12 reps, it's time to add enough weight so that you can barely do 8 again.

If you can only do 7, you can live with that. But if you can only do 6, you've added too much weight. Take a little off. The range could be 10-12, 6-9, or only 8-9 reps a muscle. Stick with those guidelines.

Want to prove me wrong? All you need to do to prove me wrong right now is just go ahead and cut your workouts down to one half of what they currently are. Drop half the sets you do or half the exercises, either way, start to do this today. With what is left, know you do not need to hold back, so go ahead and try for as many repetitions as you possibly can.

Once you see you can do more reps than you expected, tell me what happened. And don't stop. Keep at it for at least one full week. Perform half the exercise, put in twice the effort. If you like, wait until the end of the first week to drop me a line. No need to attach an apology.

This program is a bit different than what are known as medically supported but it doesn't take a Ph.D. to understand the facts (it seems to take one to overlook them though). You see, most physicians look for the answer they WANT and then gather the info they need to substantiate their theories.

It's like using a plastic fork with a metal one right in front of and insisting either will do then arguing that yours is just as good. Then it snaps. This is why many physicians spend their careers defending the contradictions people throw at them. The contradictions are the simple things that were overlooked to begin with. It's true.

How many physicians are used on a regular basis for being innovative? None. They are either local or you LIKE them as a person, but any one physician will do. And that's NO stipulation to base decisions on. That brings up another good point too. Let's use me as an example. I really and sincerely do not mind if you think I am a jerk at times.

As long as I teach you something, you learn something, and we both know I am at least honest and a step ahead of where you are right now, it doesn't matter whether you like me or not. It's not about like. It's about results. Sure, you would think a physician has a lot more education than I do but the little bit I know that they do not, THAT IS THE DIFFERENCE!

I am also sure some of you still think you know what you are talking about too and maybe you bought this book only to challenge me about my ideas. That's a good excuse but I haven't bought a fitness related book in over 10 years. I am THAT secure with what I do.

Speaking of insecurity, look yourself in the mirror right now. Are you ashamed? Are you afraid to see yourself in the mirror as you exit the shower? Have you been to the beach lately? Do you walk around like He-man thinking you are cooler than other people? Do you use plastic surgery to make up for areas you are insecure about then claim it is for 'work' related purposes or just so 'you' feel better about something? That's insecurity.

I know because I too was once insecure. I never wanted to be the skinny guy, but I was and I am glad I was. It allowed me to be the geek at one point, suffer ridicule and get picked on as a teenager. Those were life lessons. Gaining weight allowed me to hang with the 'in' crowd but you know what, I didn't change inside. Neither did they, and that was the problem. I went from being treated like 'white trash' because I was skinny to being treated like 'one of them' once I was a healthy weight.

Yes, being skinny is 'odd' but so is the idea you're gaining weight for someone else's approval instead of merely your own health purposes. To think we do anything for approval is awful. To think someone NEEDS YOUR approval is just as lame. However, if you are ready to change for yourself, and not for others, let's go!

KNOW HOW AEROBICS

One day a man somewhere between the age of 40 or 45 walking into a martial arts academy and expressed an interest in taking some lessons. He began watching the class for a little while and notices that some of the 'senior' students look very relaxed and appear to be enjoying themselves immensely, while some of the ' newer' students are straining, red faced, stressed, tense and quickly exhausted. He calls the instructor over to the viewing area and asks why there is such a dramatic difference between the two groups. He goes on to state that he has come in today because he had seen one of the guys from class over at the local gym and pointed out that this kid was in pretty good shape. "But shouldn't he be able to outlast these other guys?" he asks.

Now before I tell you what was explained to him, I would like to clarify a few things first. The Know How is not a program that is against methods of aerobic training like stationary bicycles, treadmills, stair climbers, etc. These machines and even their counter parts i.e. mountain bikes, running stadium stairs or going for a jog all have their place and there are even scientific formulas that one can use to meet goals we never could without them. I simply choose to tell this story to those of you who possibly don't see yourselves using the above-mentioned apparatus to achieve those goals.

I think many of us would like to know how else to incorporate some aerobics into our training and benefit from other activities/hobbies that we enjoy, rather than simply doing aerobics for the sake of doing them. Let's get back to the story shall we? The man who saw this other young fellow excelling on the aerobic machines at the fitness club also saw that same young guy this night run completely out of gas and become completely exhausted in a matter of minutes wrestling! It's all about 'functional' strength he was told. He looks at the instructor a little confused and says "Isn't that what the lifting of weights is for?" Yes and no.

The conversation goes on to give him an everyday example of the differences like when you go to carry your groceries out of the store. Assuming you're not too lazy and just push one of those carts, then you will notice that from your "weight training" they don't seem as heavy as they used to. You're stronger. He agrees.

However, did you also notice that after you've carried them all the way to the end of the parking lot that they did still seem ALOT heavier the further you carried them and you are now winded too? He smirks like he relates to what he is hearing. This is the difference between functional strength and aerobic conditioning!

A senior student comes over to ask something, and it became clear to both of them that the student had been working hard and that his heart rate was elevated. His deep, heavy breathing gave that away. No calculations of 220 minus your goat's age and dividing by how many eggs you eat were even necessary to arrive at the conclusion he was working hard. This student had been using EVERY muscle in his body for a wrestling session that lasted about 15 minutes or so. The coach told the visitor that by training in this particular martial art, you end up doing any sort of a combination of bends, twists, kicks, pulls, shoves, holds, pins, etc that are performed repetitiously enough to become the equivalent of doing aerobics. Not Tae Bo...

Coupling this sort of aerobic training WITH demanding exercises at a gym brings about a functional strength level that indeed exceeds that of spending hours on a stair stepper because it carries over to many of our daily activities. Yes, like carrying groceries to the car. How often in life will you be required to run for 3 hours? Not often. But those bursts of energy to do house work, carry groceries, they pop up often, but they aren't half as tough as going all out for 15 minutes at a time, are they? The instructor could see that he was looking at the class in a completely different way now.

He was beginning to understand that aerobics didn't have to be done on a bike, or a rowing machine and that doing them on a machine may not help him do the things that HE does regularly any better. There is no flexibility involved, no variation in movement… Suddenly martial arts became realistic, in a functional sort of way. Aerobics should play an important role in your life. To feel more alive, have more energy and add quality time to your schedule are reasons enough to at least cut back. Interestingly enough, there have been substantiated studies that prove deep diaphramatic or 'deep' breathing practiced regularly can actually have as much if not more effect on the cardiovascular system than running on a treadmill for 30 minutes!

Sounds strange doesn't it? If we think about why we do cardio to begin with, it is to increase the amount of oxygen that is taken into our bloodstream. Deep breathing is what rapidly increases this factor. We do aerobics just to stimulate fat loss through deeper breathing. That's all. We are forced to do this because most of us are shallow (or chest) breathers almost all the time. We need to breath into our bellies, our diaphragms, if we want our lungs to really fill up and get much needed oxygen into our cells. Our fast paced, high stress, modern lives have led us to shallow breathing instead of doing what we did as babies. We started out breathing so deep our bellies expanded. What happened along the way that we stopped?

I'm not trying to sell a deep breathing course. I am suggesting you get a singing coach though. Just joking. Sort of. This is where I learned to apply the techniques so you know… What I am trying to do is open up your eyes to the truth about aerobics. Whether you would like to take a martial arts class, or maybe even play golf then that's what you should do! But in the golf example, golf alone won't raise your heart rate enough or supply you with enough oxygen to give you the healthful results you're after. However, having the combination of golf AND something that induces deep breathing will!

And hopefully you KEEP deep breathing even when you're NOT exercising…. You weight lift for strength. You perform cardio for endurance. We do both of these things so we continue to enjoy doing 'everyday' things and perhaps to give us the desired results in tone or fat loss. Either way, you are much more apt to make any form of exercise a long term part of your lifestyle if you can do something you enjoy at the SAME TIME. So what does all this mean to you? Well, I'm hoping that you realize that you don't have to seek high tech equipment or expensive memberships to achieve your health goals.

You can join a martial arts class or find something similar you can do right in your own home! It takes a whole lot less time and money than what you think and I bet my bottom dollar that it can be a whole lot more fun than you expect! The funny thing is, now that I practice this, I have cut to 15 minutes instead of 3 times that and I am much leaner, healthier, fuller, and stronger than ever before. I am not kidding when I say I am in better shape and carry less fat than when I weighed 50 pounds lighter. It's amazing. And I am the benefits roll over into all areas of my life. Sure, you may be a lady looking to lose maybe 10, 20 or 50 pounds instead of gaining muscle.

But it's all relative. Although you need aerobic exercise to strengthen your heart, lungs, and veins in order to pump nutrients to your muscles and toxins out of your system, it is still NOT the best way to lose body fat. No matter what you believe or how you think that others you admire train, I am here to tell you that you must first diet right, and then second, weight lift with a brief but intense bout of cardio after each session if you want to look your best.

This limited amount of aerobics is enough to increase your vital capacity (the useable portion of your lungs) if you really do give it your all. The problem is, most people do not know how hard is hard enough to achieve visible results.

The experts say you know you are working hard enough if you use the figure found by deducting your age from 220 and multiplying that by .7 (it determines the heart rate in beats per minute required for proper cardiovascular work). If you are 30, it doesn't matter if you weigh 100 or 800 pounds, you will deduct 30 from 220 which is 190 and multiplying that by .7 and get 133. So if you are anywhere around 133 beats a minute, you're 'in the zone' for fat loss. But what if you are 90 years old? Well, 220 - 90 = 130 x .7 = 90 beats a minute maximum...

I say just get off your butt, weight train for 20 minutes, check and see if this doesn't double your resting heart rate. If not, that's alright, see if you are at least working hard enough to breath heavy without gasping for air. If so, great, if not, then aerobics are not going to help you burn fat.

After 15 minutes of, as I like to say, "Huff and Puff", leave. You're done. And the best aerobic machines to use for this are recumbent cycles and rowing machines in my opinion. Ladies, stair masters do work your butt, however they also lead to large calves (unattractive) and so does walking on a treadmill at an incline (or walking too fast without actually jogging). Keep in mind, as time progresses and weeks pass, you will be able to increase the intensity of your aerobic exercise (by walking faster, rowing faster, riding faster), but once you can jog, either move to another exercise or start jogging. In other words, you must strive to 'travel' further in the same time frame, every session, if you want to keep burning fat.

What if you're 90? What if you have high blood pressure? F.Y.I. The American Heart Association says blood pressure above 140mm Hg systolic and 90mm Hg diastolic is high and 120 'over' 70 is what's considered healthy. Systolic is the amount of pressure against your artery walls during the heart's contraction and diastolic is the pressure or ease thereof during the heart's relaxation period between beats.

Aerobics will elevate your blood pressure a bit but this is safe because it's under limited and controlled durations. Think of it as doing something to open up clogged drains and allowing for clearer 'breathing' passages while at rest. The research to confirm this was performed by testing the four measures of cardiovascular health in both athletic clientele and seniors. The areas studied were heart rate, maximum oxygen uptake, stroke volume, and ejection fraction. The most enhanced individual progress reported clinically came from short bursts of exercise, not continual aerobic movement. What does this mean? Ever lost your breath after only a few sets of weights? That was your aerobic pathway taking over after the an-aerobic pathway (weight lifting) ended.

Your body started building its cardiovascularity without you actually doing anything 'aerobic'. Go figure. Notice what happens the next time you lift a weight or start breathing heavy during a martial arts class or carrying groceries. It's all the same. Do you understand what I am getting at? You do not need a lot of aerobics in your life to make progress. What type of aerobics you choose should be selected based upon what will allow you to perform greater intensity from session to session and also allows for enough variety you can keep from being bored. What do I do?

Sometimes I run. Sometimes I do sprints. Sometimes I ride a bike. But twice a week I practice martial arts of course. Some of you think I mean that I take Tae Bo or use video cassettes. No, that's not it. Remember what I do for a living? I own a martial arts studio. So for 15 minutes after I am depleted from lifting weights, I hit the heavy bag, kick it or grapple with a stronger student. If Billy Blanks got you off your butt and his tapes are what motivated you to exercise, God bless him. But if you do his or any other form of cardio for more than 20 minutes until you're dropped your fat down, you are defeating the purpose. Look at all the fat aerobic instructors and women who never lose a pound if you do not believe me.

Too much cardio eats away at your muscle. Not eating right doesn't make matters better. In fact, if you limit your cardio to 15 minutes after weights, I honestly feel you can add a few sessions on the side at 20 minutes each every week and be just fine. I do not encourage this at first because I believe you will misunderstand what that means and abuse the privilege, but I think you understand. It is alright to do 2 or 3 sessions of aerobics a week extra if you do not exceed 20 minutes a session, if you have a protein meal before hand, and if you are at least down to those last 10 to 15 pounds of fat to burn.

I have already mentioned this. Until then, stick to the rules, please. You really do not need more. Unless your heart rate is up to 50% of your max heart rate (which is also achieved through weight training) and you have depleted your glycogen (muscle energy) levels without losing muscle (through weight training too) aerobics are not going to help you burn anyhow. Remember when you first started running or riding a bike? You only went so far for the longest time, like a mile at the most, but one day, ONE DAY, out of nowhere, you decided to keep going and actually was able to keep going further than expected? Say for 6 or 10 or maybe more miles?

What gives? You didn't train for that. You only trained for a mile at a shot. All you need is a little conditioning to be capable of a lot of activity believe it or not. Aerobics only do 'so much' for you. Weight training does the rest. If we train hard for short bursts, the conditioning will allow for longer ones almost automatically. And again, I like Billy Blanks. He is motivating. I like Bruce Lee too. But I do not pretend martial arts aerobics will make me into a martial artist nor allow me to understand what it is like to defend myself if necessary. Many classes I have taken in the past were classes of just kicks, punches, combinations, abdominal exercises and maybe some other stuff. It can be grueling and tiring. Problem is, I remember many students not getting into better shape taking the classes and others that just couldn't last a full hour long session.

We know that was partially due to their not eating right and weight training. But like myself, at one point, it was also due to doing too much aerobic oriented work. Being able to last an hour long of aerobics doesn't necessarily mean you are better conditioned. I know plenty of marathon runners that spend 9 months of the year sick as dogs. Nor do aerobics teach you to defend yourselves.

A lot of ladies take Tae Bo and some of you have bought the videos thinking what you learn will protect you from a purse snatcher or allow you to stand up for your lady in a bar. Not true. Yes, I want you to look at martial arts as aerobic, but I do not want you to look at aerobics as martial arts. It is my intention to help those of you who want variety in your aerobics to think of yourselves as potential students of the martial arts. Through just a little training, 15 minutes, 3 days a week, maybe even only 2, we can teach you how to sharpen and hone the natural tools you didn't even know you had. This is important because like it or not, odds are, all of us at one time or another will be attacked.

Through just 15 minutes of work after each weight training session spent either with a partner or a punching bag, you may be more than able to walk away from that attack standing tall. No one wants to mess with someone who at least knows one or two moves to defend themselves. They haven't a clue what else is in your arsenal, so most often, they back off rather than push the issue. You do not have to look like Arnold, nor have the skills of Jackie Chan. But you should be able to get through a weight training session and then 12 minutes of punches and kicks without getting too winded if you expect to protect yourself.

No attack will ever last 40 minutes, so brief and quick is key here. If you can make it through a training session that's 30 minutes total, you can make it through a purse snatcher or drunken buffoon attack. To accomplish this, you must practice techniques that you have seen work or are proven to be the most beneficial.

262   **www.ExerciseAndNutritionTheTruth.com**

Once you have studied and rehearsed them to a point they are easy, learn others. I also recommend getting instruction in boxing. Learn to use a speed bag. There is nothing like hitting the speed bag after a workout. Besides, your opponent may be an out of work boxer. You do not necessarily need to know ring strategy, but learning how to use your hands for a real fighting situation may come important. Knocking a bag around like Rocky Balboa can be quite cardiovascular. You'll see once you try it. Kicking and punching the air is not true preparation for self defense. You need to actually strike something or have a friend to beat on (just kidding, don't try to hurt someone). If you are looking into getting a heavy bag for your home to practice with, get one that hangs low around your shin level and yet is tall enough that it's around 6 foot high.

Eventually you will move up to rehearsing knee and shin blows. Hey, an opponent on the street may be a pro at kickboxing! I do not want you paranoid that you're being stalked or there is always a chance you may be attacked, but that is how people get hurt. They aren't prepared if they are. My next suggestion here is that you look into ground fighting, grappling, wrestling or Gracie Barra Jiu Jitsu. It will come as quite a surprise as to how much fat you will lose learning to go one on one with an attacker, how confident you will become in your everyday life and how much you will learn to respect others by learning and rehearsing these arts 15 minutes, 3 times a week. Do not become fascinated by belts and competitions.

On the street, there isn't time to find out what rank the opponent is nor see if the referee is watching to keep them from getting too rough. Your self-protection rests in your own hands. There are a thousand different moves and techniques and a million different ways of applying them. Every situation and instructor is going to be different. The moves or techniques that you use against a short fighter, may not work against a taller fighter, or a thinner opponent as it would a fatter, men vs. women and vice versa.

Your instructor will teach you what they feel is most beneficial but you may let them know you really are looking for something specific. No matter the situation, you must always consider the possibility that a trip to the store, to the gym, the bank or worse, sleeping at home, may lead to an attack by a stranger or someone we previously trusted. It is better to be prepared and not have to use your skills, rather than to need skills and not have any! Here are a few things to keep in mind when training to defend yourself:

Keep your eyes open and pay attention to your opponent's moves. Attack directly, strike as though you will only need to strike once but follow through with as many more blows as necessary. That will either give the attacker second thoughts or you're gonna successfully stop them! Besides that, know the ground, the area, and even the direction of the sun and wind around you. I wouldn't throw kicks on a wet surface. I wouldn't stand with my face in the wind or sun because it's blinding. Circle the opponent to let the wind blow or sun shine on them instead. Got a good idea of what you need to do now?

Ladies, try this. It will benefit you. Besides, stair masters do not work your butt, they lead to large calves (unattractive) and so does walking on an incline (or walking too fast) on a treadmill. Speaking of which, if you are able to increase the intensity of the exercise (by walking faster, rowing faster, riding faster) you better if you want to keep burning fat, but the hard core 10 to 15 minute duration rule must never be exceeded. Your body will start burning the glucose stored as glycogen (body starch) in your muscles and liver if you do. If I taught you today that you need only short aerobic training to get results, that variety is OK and that learning to defend yourself not only makes sense but it can be substituted for cardio work a few times a week, then my job is done.

For more on martial arts. visit: MartialArtsChampions.com

STRETCHING

Here is something taken directly from the narration of the exercise videos I filmed for QVC. Use them as prescribed after you have worked the muscles, not before, for reasons already discussed.

Hamstring Stretch: One heel on a platform one foot or so off the ground. Keep that leg straight and toes pointed towards you as you squat down a little bit on your other leg. Keep both hips equally pivoted forward and your shoulders back. I do not recommend using anything higher than knee level. Hold for 20 seconds each leg and VIOLA! Hamstrings are stretched!

Lower Back Stretch: Sit down on your knees on the floor. Lean forward. Optimally your knees should be spread apart so that you can more easily get your ribs toward the floor. Really stick your rump back and try to press your chest onto the floor as you reach as far forward as possible with your hands. Do not allow your butt to leave your feet. Hold for 20 seconds.

Glute Stretch: Take a seat on the floor. Pull one knee up to your chest and hold that same legs foot up higher. Where you place your hands is of utter importance. Sitting up straight, one hand pulls the inside of your knee to the center of your chest from under the backside of your upper leg while the other hand is under your ankle not pulling in but holding that foot up. Your knee is pulled into the center of your chest as your other foot is held 6 inches higher than your knee is. Try holding for 20 seconds each leg.

Thigh Stretch: Find a rack or platform a little lower than your butt and place the top of your foot and toes on it behind you. Stand close enough to put your heel on your butt. Squat down on the other leg while leaning your shoulders back. You want the other knee joint farther back than the hip joint as you squat downward.

Feel it on the entire front of the leg. Hold for 20 seconds. Repeat on other leg.

Ab, Lat, And Tricep Stretch: This one is a little confusing. Stand placing your weight on one foot. Cross the other foot behind you. Raise your arm overhead, bend that elbow, point it to the sky and place your thumb to your spine behind your neck. With the other hand, grasp your elbow, pull it to the opposite side and lean with it bending yourself kind of in half. Feel this in the back of your upper arm, armpit, ribs and stomach. Hold for twenty seconds each side. This is easier than it sounds. Stand placing most of your weight on one foot. Cross the other behind you. Reach overhead bending it at the elbow. Place your thumb on your spine. Grasp that elbow with the opposing hand and pull with the other arm in the opposite direction. When pulling to the side, lean into it enough to make yourself feel like a pretzel. Push the hip out and pull the elbow over to really stretch the AB's hard. Do 20 seconds both sides. If you use a partner to assist, one of your partner's hands should be on your shoulder as their other hand pulls your elbow back towards them a little bit and then across and behind you towards the other side of your body. Repeat with other arm as well.

Rack Lat Stretch: Put your hands close together on a rack about waist height. Do not bounce!!! Find as sturdy rack as possible to use. Put your feet close to or on the bottom of this rack. Hang your butt down low, keep your legs straight, pull with straight arms, push with your feet a bit but keep your butt off the floor. Hold for 20 seconds before slowly rising back up. You know, you should always stretch your muscles after working them.

Shoulder And Bicep Stretch: Do you have an assistant? Have your partner stand behind you holding your wrists and palms downward and arms extended behind you. Rotate your shoulder blades and elbows backward and squat downward. Stay low, leaning a little forward for 20 seconds.

Works best if your partner actually raises your hands a little higher for you. Hands close together, palms down, that's the key.

Chest Stretch Seconds: Stand by an upright rack or wall with your palm, forearm, and elbow firmly against that fixture. Position your elbow at shoulder height. Have your elbow only as high as your shoulder the entire time and turn your body away from your arm which remains firm against the wall. The aim is to lean a little forward while the arm props you back. Hold for 20 seconds. Repeat for other side.

Neck Stretch: With your hands acting as a hook, push into the floor with your feet. This is not that difficult, find a rack that is about knee level and you can clasp your hands onto because once you grasp this rack you must not so much pull on it but push downward with your feet into the floor. While holding your chin into your chest and your hands acting as that hook, it is then that you push into the floor with your feet as the stretch is felt across the back of your shoulders and neck. 20 seconds.

Do you really need to stretch?

Stretching is useful for both injury prevention and injury treatment. For the purposes of this discussion I will concentrate on prevention. If done properly, stretching increases flexibility and this directly translates into reduced risk of injury. The reason is that a muscle/tendon group with a greater range of motion passively, will be less likely to experience tears when used actively.

Stretching is also thought to improve recovery and may enhance athletic performance. The latter has not been fully agreed upon in the medical literature, but improved biomechanical efficiency has been suggested as an explanation. Additionally, increased flexibility of the neck, shoulders and upper back may improve respiratory function.

HOME GYMS SELECTING A HOME GYM

I know that most of you believe in me and I have your trust. However, there are others who may read this and feel differently due to the point I want to get across. If this is you, I want to take this moment to help you clearly understand that I will not try to force you or anyone else to follow my advice nor any other program for that matter. It makes no difference to me whether what you think is right is actually 'right' or wrong. I will however attempt to pass along to you what I know in a sincere effort to let the facts be known regardless. So let me explain why this chapter is so important.

There are 4 types of fitness equipment or resistance used to choose from when creating a new routine or setting up a workout that suits your needs. The first is constant resistance exercise equipment. This is the type of stuff where throughout the entire movement, the weight seems to remain the same (you'll understand what this means in a second). The second is variable resistance technology. This is the type of equipment where the resistance or feel of the weight seems to change at some points (like with Nautilus equipment where it gets harder to lift the weight the closer to the muscular contraction point you get).

The third type of resistance is static, or isometric exercise. This is the type of movement where there is no actual movement up or down at all with the exception of the pushing or pulling effect itself you use to cause the muscle to contract. Last but not least we have accommodating resistance. This form of exercise is the type where both the weight and the speed are easily controlled by the lifter. You cannot perform them all at once, nor should you try to, especially all in one session. You probably don't have access to all the different machine types to do so even if you wanted to. Despite machines being easier and safer to use that barbells and dumb bells in most cases, you cannot forgo free style weights for the machines.

While machines isolate your muscles better than barbells or dumbbells, without barbells, you are never going to fully develop your co-ordination skills, strength nor burn the fat you want to. Why? Because you need to use all different forms of resistance and no routine is good unless it is first run it's course and then restructured for variety.

If you really want to reach your full potential, you will use a little of anything and everything you can get your hands on to train with. Where do you begin? Just pick one. If I had to pick, I would probably select a different technology depending the muscle. Each muscle reacts better or best depending on what one we are discussing. I might say that something like the original Nautilus machines with their variable resistances. If I hadn't much of a choice, ANYTHING WILL DO. Just lift something!

Have you seen any of those fitness infomercials on late night television? The ones where all you need is to make three easy payments and you will soon have the perfect body of your dreams using their wonderful toys. If that's true, then why don't you or anyone else have the body of their dreams using this junk? And why do only washed up TV stars, not current or movie stars, hawk that crap? Career INTEGRITY.

Keep in mind, no matter who is endorsing those products on TV, anything that works only one muscle or offers little resistance, isn't worth wasting your time on. In fact, the woman who supposedly developed the first abdominal curler or cruncher (or whatever it was) ever sold on modern TV bragged to us one day that her product was pure junk and that she never even used it. She was a member of my gym at the time QVC sold her junk! Millions of Americans buy home gym equipment every year. I am sure you know someone who has something off TV and does NOT use it! Be it one piece of equipment or many, nothing works unless it offers more than one exercise and one of the top 4 forms of resistance. I realize having a gym membership doesn't guarantee you'll exercise either. Some of us lack the time.

And the gyms themselves are not exactly jumping through hoops for you to attend either. They like the club being empty because they can sell more memberships that way. Besides, they already have your cash, monthly credit card or automatic debit payment anyways.

If you aren't wasting the investment, a gym membership is good since you get to use all the different equipment that obviously can't fit in your house but I do not always feel like nor have the opportunity to attend. I am NOT attacking gyms. I travel, I get overloaded with work, and who knows your reasoning? I have a solution to all of this. Go to the gym when you can, say twice a week, then use an affordable, total body home gym on another day or whenever you can't get to the gym. EVEN WHEN YOU TRAVEL. What gym fits in your purse or is no bigger than a folded t-shirts?

You have probably seen the Bodylastics product on QVC alongside the crap I wouldn't touch with a ten foot pole. It is the elastic band home gym kit put together by my good friend Blake Kassel. He is not just the owner of the Bodylastics company and I am not just an endorser, but we are both proud users. And he has become such a good friend of mine that he actually mentioned Don Lemmon's KNOW HOW briefly in his last QVC appearance! If you haven't personally heard of him, that's alright. Grab some water, and check this out. The Bodylastics kit is something similar to the elastic bands used in aerobics classes except these ones have tension equal anywhere from 5 to 100's of pounds in my favorite, VARIABLE resistance! No kidding. This home gym is so innovative that it has been featured in numerous national publications like Glamour, New Woman, Delta Sky, Woman's World, Jane, Men's Exercise, Prevention, You Gotta Read This and Essence magazines. What at first appears to be nothing more than a simple set of 4 rubber bands with handles is really something that professional athletes, personal trainers and bodybuilders use too.

What you have here is a complete barbell set or what's close to a complete fitness center membership all in one 2 pound bag. The only difference is that this gym doesn't have anyone waiting in line ahead of you and you won't need to clear an entire garage out to make room for it. And for less than the cost of one month at any health club, Men, Women, Children, the Elderly, and the Athletic, can all use this anytime, and anywhere. It fits in a suitcase or a purse and all you need is the space around you at arms length to use it. Our friends in Japan, where living spaces are quite limited, really seem to love us for that!

I know that personally, I regret leaving home for business trips because that means I must actually go out and find a gym because hotels rarely have anything worth using and the process is such a pain in the neck. I have spent way too much time looking for the local gyms, calling them one by one for directions, and you know the routine.... Getting ready, driving there, finding parking, signing in, waiting for a guest tour, making my way around the naked people hanging out in the locker room for no apparent reason, finally getting to work out, only to wait in line for the equipment, then trying to get back to the hotel or home again ... It's a 4 hour process for a 30 minute workout that I just don't have time for.

I have traveled by car and by plane across the United States so many times I can't even assume to remember how often that I have experienced headaches with owners, people behind the counter thinking they have power for a change or salespeople that really ought to be trying to sell local customers. There is one gym that sticks out in my mind because they treated me like I was a member for years each time I passed through. That gym is called Popeye's and it is located in Topeka, Kansas. I am not kidding when I say that most everywhere else I have been I felt like I was asking people if I could pull their teeth rather than paying them to use their clubs. These days, I do not even bother. I use my Bodylastics kit.

Friends of mine use Bodylastics to warm themselves up before they go on stage, doing a photo shoot, looking pumped up for a date or even heading out on to the playing field to warm up. Imagine how much of a benefit it is not to lug dumbbells around with you everywhere from now on for these things. I like the kit so much I had Blake send me extra straps so I can work up to an amazing 500 pounds of resistance on some of my favorite movements.... Can you picture this? I can take a broom stick, slide it through the handles, place the stick across my back, and suddenly I am squatting hundreds of pounds and there's no weight to rack or unrack afterwards! By simply using any given number of the four different sized elastic bands, the kit accommodates almost all of the various levels of strength you could imagine between a pro wrestler and a grandparent.

I used to be a bodybuilder. My close friends still are or have become pro athletes. None of us could do a complete curl or a squat using the entire four bands for 10 reps on our first attempt. A few of us couldn't do all 4 bands at all on most movements. That's a lot of resistance. And I am a pretty strong guy! Drop a couple bands and seconds later, your father can start to use them. The unique clip system attached to both ends of the bands is what allows you to vary the resistance or weight lifted so quick. And because of the handles, there are so many exercises you can perform with these things. Not only does each muscle group have several choices of exercise, but by varying the number of bands, you can get the maximum stimulus for each without ever feeling under-worked or over-worked at any level you have achieved.

Other elastic sets come with either both handles permanently attached to one elastic (which doesn't allow you to use more than one band), or you are forced to adjust the resistance level by rolling up the rubber. This causes wobbling, a disruption of the body's natural movement and more often than not, slippage and injury. Imagine what happens if the bands unravel. WHAP! Right in the face!

I couldn't let my kid or grand mother use something like that. This is something I believe makes this better than Bowflex and Soloflex combined. Trust me, you don't need bulky equipment to get into shape. You simply need something that adds resistance to your exercise. Something that makes working against gravity a little tougher. The Bodylastics home gym can effectively do all of the above for right around $40.00 You read that right. You are about to not only save hundreds if not thousands of dollars on exercise equipment, but you can even get this product for less than the official Bodylastics website and QVC charges.

It was proven years ago that the only way to change the shape or appearance of your body is to make your muscles tone. The only way to do that is to make them stronger. To gain strength, a muscle must lengthen (eccentric movement) and shorten (concentric contraction) against some form of resistance. But your muscles are blind. They do not know, nor care, if you are curling a barbell, a dumbbell or a machine. They only know that you are working against some sort of resistance and variable resistance is best, but you need something besides a machine to build co-ordination and skill at the same time. As long as this is met and it is something heavy enough for you to feel the stress, this resistance can come in the form of Bodylastics or bricks. It doesn't matter. Bricks unfortunately cannot allow for the following exercises:

Pushups (yes, pushups, but now they can be performed with as much resistance as bench presses), chest flyes (normally done with dumbbells), crossovers (without cables), side lateral shoulder raises (without dumbbells or a machine), front shoulder raises (ditto), front and rear military presses (no barbell needed), lat pull downs, pullovers, bent over rows, seated rows, shrugs, rear pull downs, squats, lunges, hip extensions, leg extensions, deadlifts, hamstring curls, calf raises, biceps curls, preacher curls, overhead triceps extensions, kickbacks, tricep pushdowns, situps, crunches (better than any ab roller), hyperextensions, inclined movements, forearm exercises and MORE...

I even figured out how to leg presses with these things. What's even more important to point out besides variety is the fact you can perform all movements through a complete range of motion. I think I made it clear how vital that is to developing quick and permanent results over the years.

The one concern we have is that you go out and try to overstretch the elastics. The bands carry an extensive warranty. If they snap, we replace them. But do not think for a second that if it's clear you are playing tug of war with them from across the room or using the bands to strap down furniture on a truck that it won't result in weakening and/or breakage.

So the truth of the matter is that you must decide, is it worth having a kit like this that costs around $40 to replace the gym on the days you haven't access to the club? Yes it is. But then again, maybe you haven't anything to train on at home to begin with and you are considering other options. Whatever equipment interests you, it must still meet the demands of allowing for progression. If you cannot add weight to an exercise when you need to or cannot move up the speed on a cardio machine fast enough to keep up with your conditioning, you're in trouble. Our entire lives are based on trying for more and more. Do not forget this fact. The only other piece of home gym equipment I use is a stationary bike. It cost me a few hundred dollars and it's a bike that's been on the market for over 30 years. I like it.

I do not recommend or endorse any particular brand name or type of equipment unless I like it. I do not know how much space you have to work with so I will leave it at that. As far as health club equipment, I love Med-x, Hammer Strength, Nautilus, barbells, dumbbells and other properly built pieces of equipment that come in all sorts of shapes and sizes. I like aerobic rowing machines and bikes more than I like treadmills and stair climbers. But I haven't room for all of them at home, in fact most of them, and I do not always feel like fighting traffic even locally and that's why I have my little rubber band kit.

However, it's important that you do your own research and choose the items that are best for you. I've provided you with plenty of info to build upon. It's now up to you to gather more information. Check out Blake's site at Bodylastics.com

Tell the Rubber Band Man I sent you. Otherwise, drop me a line or send a check for $40 made out to BODYLASTICS and I will forward it off to him. Since moving to Hawaii, I haven't been to a gym but 3 times. This is a true story. I had to figure out what could replace the gym, excitement and exercises and had no where else to turn but Bodylastics and I am glad I did. Now, the entire 45 day body transformation I went through is chronicled at RefuseToFail.com but here is the routine I used to get what is sincerely, the best shape of my life:

Clapping, Marine style pushups.
Abdominal crunches.
Pushups with Bodylastics bands.
Isometric, hand to hand, pectoral movement.
Bodylastic rowing from a doorway.
Overhead tricep, lat pulldown, hand to hand isometrics.
Lying, ankle to ankle, leg extension/curl, isometrics.
Bodylastics bicep curls.
Bodylastics leg presses.
Bicep curl/tricep pushdown, hand to hand, isometrics.

That would be one set of each exercise every other day on the average. It doesn't seem like much but I look better than anyone else on this side of the island, I can assure you that much. Since I sit on my butt all day, I casually rode a stationary bike I bought for my patio afterwards. I actually kept track of everything I was feeling, thinking, experiencing, eating, doing and considering to do, including work and sleep and playtime with the wife in a diary. You should check out the site. It is at least worth a laugh seeing me in my undies.

CLOSING THOUGHTS

The first edition of my program was only 28 pages and left a lot of what you were craving hidden from view. It sold 25,000 copies and detailed the exact training programs and dietary routines to achieve what those you emulate have. Imagine, all you need forever in just 28 pages. Nothing else. Thanks to your demand, there is almost 20 times the amount of pages here. It wouldn't have been possible without support. Growth depends upon it.

I want to thank and say that I am forever grateful that God or whomever is up there allowed my time on Earth to overlap with so many amazing people including my wife Asia Carrera.

Asia alone has changed me in a multitude of ways as I have her. Nothing and no one is more important to me… I also thank Jason Gateman (thinkbigdesigns.com), Dave Campbell, Blake Kassel (bodylastics.com), Paul Becker, Harold Whiting, Robert Gaffney (omeganutrition.com), Tom Clark, Suzanne Clark, Randi and William Sellier (tjclarkminerals.com), Gary Augustine Warren (chhpresents.com), Harrison Khordestani, Brian Perich, Dave at FitnessMenus.com and if you were forgotten, forgive me. This list is off the top of my head after weeks of nonstop typing and just trying to think of people who have emailed me lately! This book is almost entirely dedicated to my daughter Carly in loving memory to Carly's Grand Father, Donald E. Lemmon Sr. who passed away just days short of Thanksgiving, 1994.

I would also like to thank those featured on my web site and in my exercise videos, plus the others whose testimonials have helped spread the word about my program. You've seen a lot of my friends in the fitness magazines, on pay-per-view, regular television or even the big screen. May my God or your God bless those who came before me, paving my way. If by chance I parallel anything you have tried before or anyone else's program you have read before, it is strictly by coincidence. If it is not, I will be the first to admit it.

Exercise & Nutrition... The TRUTH Book One

When I originally came up with the idea for Don Lemmon's Know How I was just getting out of the Army in 1988. That November I spent about two weeks driving up and down the East coast trying to figure out what I was going to do with my life and this book is one of the goals I set for myself. Sure, it's been fun, it looks like a huge success, and I am quite happy, but it hasn't been all smooth sailing. I began working with people one on one for the first time getting paid for it in Fayetteville, North Carolina back in 1988. It immediately became my passion. I am not sure where along the way I can say I fully honed my craft because I have always taught things no one else would. I do know that I feel I am learning something new daily and I sometimes cannot believe I now counsel people from around the World.

Since 1988, I've seen and heard it all. My transcripts have been stolen, sold, quoted and passed about illegally. I have had my articles put in magazines without credit, made and lost friends, seen business associates and (surprise) even family members come and go. It's been heart breaking, but enlightening nonetheless. You see, I have always believed in myself. At times I wanted to give up because everyone around me it seemed either wanted a piece of me they didn't deserve or they tried to keep me from moving forward, but deep inside, I always knew I shouldn't. I am, always was and will be the Know How forever more. I have lived it, breathed it, walked it, and felt that it just HAD to be brought public ever since pen went to paper. I didn't mean for it to stir so much water along its merry way that the people around me became divided, but it did. The only way to get things done, no matter how long it takes, or how hard it is to accomplish, is to JUST DO THEM FOR YOURSELF, not anyone else. And that's how most of this was accomplished. All alone, with little to no support. Sure, there are a few from start to finish that remained and there are plenty who have jumped on the coat tails since, but where we have come since the beginnings of it all has been nothing short of inspirational. Point is, you gotta 'keep on keeping on' sometimes.

Everything you do in life revolves around making choices. If it offends you that I say this, that's something within yourself you should take some time to deal with. Smile. Laugh. Enjoy. It is in you. Change your bad habits into good habits and lead by example instead of following the same old crowd from now on. Your life tomorrow is based upon whatever decision you make next. The truth lies within these words SO REMEMBER:

1. If what you're doing now is working, KEEP doing it. Don't be silly. Go, Go, Go!
2. If what you're doing now is NOT working, STOP doing it. Face reality. It doesn't work.
3. If you don't know what to do, DON'T do a thing. You may make things worse. Re-read this book.

Be GOOD. Do GOOD. And if anyone ever stands in your way, walk AROUND them NOT over them. Your physique, energy levels, and newfound health depend upon the commitment you have made today to listen to genuinely basic and common sense things I have presented. I know that when you walk into a law office you expect the people there to know law. When you go to a bar you expect the bartender to know his liquors.

You even depend upon mechanics to know their jobs well enough to work on pretty much anything with a motor in it but things couldn't possibly be further from the truth. People in all professions specialize in particular branches of their field. If your goal is to be taken prisoner by Xena the Warrior Princess or to go on a Legendary Journey with Hercules, I can't help you there. If your goal is to look your best naturally, become healthier doing and enjoy the path for a change, hey, I am your man. But you'll be surprised at how many people work in this industry that haven't a clue how to teach you these simple things. The path I took is a bit different than you have followed before, but it works, and this is why we are often referred to as The "UN" Diet! If you ever have questions, EMAIL ME.

I know you will always have valid concerns and questions. There are many things to take into consideration while making a lifelong commitment to yourself, but I have covered most of them before and to me it is second hand knowledge. I want to see your current diet and training program. No time has ever been more right than now. Especially since NO FRIEND, NO NEIGHBOR, NO EQUIPMENT, NO GYM in the World GUARANTEES that you will achieve your health and fitness goals by using their services. BUT I DO!

I am confident that I can do for you what I have already done for thousands of others. Right now you are probably thinking "Does this guy want me to make an expensive commitment to personal training or phone consultations or something?" NO! It's just the opposite. I want you to email me for FREE!

Think of how the lack of motivation to do something held you back and how depression has overwhelmed you without hope until you read this book. All you are doing is seeking help, just like you did when you purchased this program. Well, you've got it. I know you want to enhance your self-esteem, reduce the risk of illness or injury, sleep better, perform your best, look your best, be a better lover and all that. I know you want to get rid of the stress in your life. I will help you via email. Just ask.

I am so insistent on this because there are far too many people who are getting ROBBED at their gyms or health food stores by clowns who get paid $5.75 an hour for part-time work that started as a hobby but turned into a means by which to make a living! Plus, I take YOUR SUCCESS very seriously. If you fail, I do not get your referrals. And I need referrals to keep this business running. If this business fails, I cannot help you nor anyone else ever again. I want to know what time you sleep, wake up, eat, what the foods are and what measures of those foods you ingest happened to be

Telling me you had a turkey sandwich isn't enough. I want to know how much meat, veggies and bread were there. Do you drink milk or juice or soda with your meals? I know it seems trifle, but tell me about it. What were your calories? Don't know? Send what you can. We will make what we can from what you know and get you going. But don't expect me to do all the work. I want you to learn, and educate, not become dependant. I also want your referrals and I appreciate them so much that you can now receive additional copies of this book at a 50% discount by sending a check or money order with $3 to cover shipping and handling to our office in the name of your friends.

One of my better known quotes: "If you are trying to get to Pittsburgh and drive past a sign saying Vancouver is 3 miles away, you're not heading in the right direction. You could keep going around the planet aimlessly and eventually only end up back where you started (drowning in an ocean of wasted effort) or you can turn around and use your new KNOW HOW."

Is there more? Certainly! Visit any or all of my websites to learn more about Books Two and Three. Book Two gives you the truth about the personal training business and how you can either climb to the top of the field or become your own coach using programs, recipes and menus on offered previously before to private clientele. Book Three is my 90 Day Log book. You actually walk alongside of me as I make a body transformation you will only believe once you see it yourself.

Start at ExerciseAndNutritionTheTruth.com today!

BONUS SECTION:
THE LOST 1996/1997 QVC EXERCISE VIDEO TAPES

Learn The Workouts! Discover How Celebrities Lose Weight Fast.... We Are Releasing Our Official RAW Exercise Workout Video Footage... 6 Hours, 25 Workouts, Over 100 Exercises & Stretches ALL ON ONE CD!

It's 2004... What took so long? Well... I think I will save that for after you see what is on this CD!

What you now have access to is ALL THREE video shoots which include 24 workouts, over 6 hours of footage, more than 100 exercises, stretching demonstrations and further behind the scenes goodies I wouldn't dare put in print here all in one CD. The workouts are as follows (Workouts #1 and #2 are in Don Lemmon's KNOW HOW Book One, routines #3 through #20 are below and routines #21 to #25 are from the 'finished' 1996 also included for the first time ever... One of the videos in the 3 to 20 section has a BONUS #26 attached... Surprise...):

VIDEO WORKOUT #3 (features 5 exercises) - featuring Janie Tomasovich from the Miss Galaxy Competitions. The sweetest of the fitness competitors we used.

VIDEO WORKOUT #4 (features 6 exercises) - featuring Markus Daxl and Carol Semple, Mr Austria and Ms Olympia. We almost bought out Carol's contract with Metrx at the time so she could promote us without other obligation. Markus was actually a client of mine from Vegas.

VIDEO WORKOUT #5 (features 7 exercises) - featuring Matt Pollino whom entered my life in 1995 and went from 150 to 200 pounds in body weight on my program by 1997. He is now a doorman at a Hollywood night club and pursuing an acting career.

VIDEO WORKOUT #6 (features 7 exercises) - featuring The Mathesens, steel workers turned national physique committee bodybuilding champs and old friends from Ohio.

VIDEO WORKOUT #7 (features 8 exercises) - featuring Angela Wolbert Clark, Pan Am Games martial arts medallist. I actually went to high school with her.

VIDEO WORKOUT #8 (features 9 exercises) - featuring Michelle Talboo, IFBB Pro Fitness Competitor, also from Ohio and a former client.

VIDEO WORKOUT #9 (features 9 exercises) - featuring male model Brian Blazek. I can't tell you how many people thought he was Mike O'Hearn at first glance including Skip Lacour who is so jealous of me he stalks my website. I announced that Don Ross caught Skip with clenbuterol at the Muscle Mania and he never forgave me. His foot went in his mouth when he emailed Mike telling him I was using his photos without permission. What an industry folks!

VIDEO WORKOUT #10 (features 10 exercises) - featuring Artie Kaikou, Shoto Kan Karate expert and Chuck Norris look a like. Artie went from 135 to 170 on my program.

VIDEO WORKOUT #11 (features 11 exercises) - featuring Versace model Momir Sornaz. Nice guy. Reminded me a lot of another good friend Eric Drury who was my training partner back in 1994 and is discussed at length in Don Lemmon's KNOW HOW Book Two.

VIDEO WORKOUT #12 (features 11 exercises) - featuring Theresa Hessler the one time Italian Fitness Champion. This girl was the worst to work with. She lied, she meddled, she did all she could to ruin everyone's time and after all those hours of consultation I gave her and her boyfriend, that's the thanks I get?

VIDEO WORKOUT #13 (features 11 exercises) – featuring Matt Pollino AKA Tiger The Martial Artist again.

VIDEO WORKOUT #14 (features 12 exercises) - featuring Susie Curry, the all time favorite at the Ms Fitness International. Susie was fun, unfortunately she got caught up in Hessler's games.

VIDEO WORKOUT #15 (features 12 exercises) - featuring Dale Tomita... The always popular Ms Fitness World from Hawaii. She was the other DIVA that tried to ruin one of the shoots.

VIDEO WORKOUT #16 (features 12 exercises) - featuring Eric Bergman. Eric's older brother and I introduced him to weightlifting. MY how he HAS grown.

VIDEO WORKOUT #17 (features 12 exercises) - featuring Karen Hulse, Ms World. Karen took a few gymnastic lessons that weekend from Matt Pollino... A real joy.

VIDEO WORKOUT #18 (features 13 exercises) - featuring Danny Weigand, the Jr USA Champion! If anyone supplied comic relief, it would be this guy!

VIDEO WORKOUT #19 (features 15 exercises) - featuring World Toughman Champion Ray Hammond. I will never forget Ray when he came to the shoot. My friend's two kids, ages 10 and 8, looked up at Ray with that lion's mane hair, 240 pounds of muscle and asked "Who are you sir?" Ray replied, "I am the TOUGHEST MAN IN THE WORLD little guys," as he reached to shake their tiny hands. They trembled with glee thinking he was Conan.

VIDEO WORKOUT #20 (features 20 exercises) - featuring Ericca Kern, Miss North America. FYI: Our company runs Ericca's official website....

VIDEO WORKOUTS #21 through #25 (#26 is hidden in one of the above)... These final routines demonstrate and explain almost all the exercises you will ever need. Ranging from 11 to 14 movements each, dozens of stretching techniques... I could easily be charging double what I do for this presentation alone... However... You can now....

So what is the story behind the "Don Lemmon" QVC Videos? To make a long story short, yeah, like I know how to do that, back in 1996 I came up with the idea to film some exercise videos using the most popular of my clientele. At first, being in Las Vegas, I planned on using clients that were part of various existing video projects like Body By Jake, martial arts aerobic instructors, and trainers seen in some of those home gym infomercials.

Unfortunately, my videos just weren't coming together. Too few people wanted the world to know I was to credit for their appearances instead of they having the KNOW HOW. I suppose that meant their clients would pay to have me train them instead or something... Others were afraid of losing clientele or endorsement contracts. Backed into a corner, I had to think of something quick. I had interested parties from television who wanted to 'sell' me but no product to offer.

Distraught, I flew home to Ohio for a break. During my stay I made some calls then drove an hour to Pittsburgh to meet with the manager of one of my clients. I got a good feeling from him so I told him more about the project than I expected and he offered further assistance. His name was J.M. Manion and in the lapse of a day, he set up my shooting to commence at his father Jim Manion's private gym a few months down the road. This worked out well in my mind as it is cheaper to fly people to Ohio than it is Vegas and I was also just a few hours from the television station headquarters that was supposed to air my goods when completed. We all win with this new path and not only that, but the location was owned by the Vice President of the organization that made Arnold Schwartzenegger a name...

Well, as they say, not all things are as easy as they first seem. Things went almost horribly wrong at that shoot and I should have learned my lesson that October. Backing out was not an option, myself and several of the video stars had plans to attend one of the largest fitness convention in the USA that following week. Here we are at the Dallas NPC Nationals... Catering to over inflated egos, people who weren't prepared to shoot on time... Editors who didn't do or seem to understand what was asked... Delays by people who didn't get their part of the project ready on schedule... People trying to get double paid... My accountant stuffing money where it was supposed to go... Gold diggers... Oh, the madness...

The way I see it now, since it was 1996 after all, despite the obvious glitches here and there, additional home styled guerilla editing, having a crew that was essentially doing something they had never experienced before and a lot of guests on the set getting in the way that were uninvited, I am surprised, and somewhat proud to say, there was a lot of cool footage captured despite after all. Sifting through everything I have, I may complain but in all honesty, I really enjoyed the laughs over things like one of the fitness champions calling a chest exercise a shoulder routine... Reliving the joking around those of us did that knew our jobs.... In fact, I would love to offer these exercise videos free so you can share in the fun and to get them out to the public as fast as possible to show how far ahead of my time this project was, however... I can't do that. I can offer them at a fair price though, and here is why....

I PRACTICALLY LOST THE SHIRT OFF MY BACK HERE

It is true. I came from Vegas to Ohio with money from personal training after giving up my quest to become a licensed physician (too many politics, needed a little more school, you know how it goes.... and with a dangling carrot of book sales instead of day to day office work... I grabbed the carrot...).

Once I figured up how much the shoot, editing, flying people in, paying them for taking off work (yes, your heroes have real jobs, they aren't rich from being in magazines, movies or on TV)... Paying for this, or that, I fell short and borrowed money from my accountant who later claimed she put in more than she had. While she figured this would make her more money, all it did was convince the others involved that they should charge more if someone else was getting more.... Which they weren't and I am sure I will go on about this in a bit... Let me get to the lighter side of things. What I am making available is still worth it's weight in gold...

If you listen closely to the advice given during any particular training session (over 2 dozen of them are on this CD), you will not only discover how much I was able to teach some of the supposedly knowledgeable clients featured but you will also recognize how I cleverly geared things towards not only the seasoned pro but beginners as well.

"This particular video product is a gem. With the first 5 routines alone, which feature the best editing, soundtrack and voice overs out of all 25 workouts, you get more advice than any other book on exercise ever read... Including MINE." ~ DON LEMMON, 2004

For a long time I felt it was too bad these tapes never got an official release on a widespread level but then again, I might not be able to offer what I am today if we did hit the networks. I wouldn't have went to the net on my own, ran my own sites, published my own books and remained so up front and personal with you. Could you imagine a Don Lemmon website where I didn't answer my own mail? Contact my own clients? It would NOT be the same...

And these videos are not any different than what my site offers... Something unique... So what are these videos like?

First thing is first, my exercise videos are nothing like the Tae Bo, Tai Chi, Tony Little or Tony Horton workout videos also available online. I do not hire actresses to pretend they are excited over my program. I am not a bloated slob and I do practice what I preach. However, I also give you the goods without frills... Aaah, no frills.... It's all raw and unedited for the most part, showing how human and silly we all are behind the scenes... I had a better time during these film shoots than it sounds when I discuss the people involved who failed me. But I can whine a little, I have earned it...

I think you can see with all the success I have had... 2 KNOW HOW Books, 2 more coming this year along with a Personal Training/Medical Certification program, 5 personally formulated supplements, 12 novels, and so much more coming (including a family with a famous woman that I adore)... I think you know I am completely happy with my life and when I complain about this project and a few of those involved, it is with reason. Don't believe me? That is fine because I have included a number of behind the scenes shots from the filming so you could see this industry isn't all fun and games and your stars aren't always perfectly behaved despite their pristine images! And there is a lot of footage to share. SIX HOURS worth...

You see, we did three shoots. The first one was in October of 1996 and it was practically a waste since the start. Oh, the footage is amazing really, the advice was beyond what anyone is offering to this day... The editing is just not what I wanted and I found myself spending so much time teaching half the stars to exercise correctly during filming that we did not get all we set out to shoot. So it goes? Sure, if your set is full of complicated people... People who do not read the script before shooting... Some of the problems I can chalk up to fate or coincidence. But some things were just plain inexcusable... Like the night before the second filming in May of 1997... We spent until 4 a.m. chasing down a stolen car. We ended up having both the local authorities AND the FBI involved. MAN, was THAT a riot...

I wish I could tell you more but two of the people hired let themselves get scammed by a couple of fans... Back to the first shoot....

The first video on the CD is the original QVC Video of 1996. It features Lee Apperson (Mr America, a true professional, seen in this photo with a 400 pound client who came to the shoot), Theresa Hessler (who was a phone consultation client with her boyfriend at the time and also the winner of Italy's Fitness title), Dr Steven Novicky (an Ohio physician), Michelle Ralabate (NPC female bodybuilding champion who was also on my first book cover), Danny Weigand (the funniest man to ever win the Mr USA title), Janie Tomasovich (a Pittsburgh nurse and competitor in the Ms Galaxy), and then Matthew Pollino and his completely meddling girlfriend who claimed to be a showgirl but proved to be a stripper, Angela Villone. Matthew liked to call himself Tiger back then. He is a talented martial artist...

She was, well, trouble... The net result of that shoot was 5 workouts included on this video CD. They each show one or two movements demonstrated by all the stars and includes both warmups, stretching and cooldowns. The audio track was recorded by two of Ohio's most popular radio show hosts and the music soundtrack provided by several artists that graced the airwaves when the footage was shot. All friends of mine and thank God, that cut the cost back a bit. And I needed that. After the editor doubling his fees, after half the stars not doing what was asked, losing footage, accountants scamming me, I was going broke. Right when I was about to give up, I surprisingly was offered assistance to help shoot more footage and patch everything up. With this help, I scheduled another two shoots in May of 1997 with the intention of having at least double the product once completed. Having double the footage and three times the amount of stars then in the cast, I was able to secure sponsors like BALANCE Bars (before they became junk food bars), Ostrim (the ostrich meat snacks, sort of like Slim Jim's...) and the ISSA (International Sports Sciences Association).

And so it goes... In the second set of exercise videos, also shot in Pittsburgh, we certainly had more diva behavior but we also had a lot more fun. In fact, I have included a clip of Janie Tomasovich and myself playfully arguing over how to perform a calf raise followed by one of the body builders Eric Bergman offering her an Ostrim ostrich meat stick snack (which she seemed disgusted about and refused), just for kicks... Things like this show we are all human and not cartoons... I think that same bodybuilder stole a whole box of those treats from me over the weekend... Matt Pollino was in this second video again too. He often questioned what part of the ostrich those sticks were made from. Food for thought? Nah! They're good!

Also in the cast besides Janie, Eric Bergman (a friend since high school who used to brag these were HIS videos so he could pick up women, silly guy) and Matt Pollino are Mr. Austria Markus Daxl (a nearly 300 pound bodybuilding client of mine from Las Vegas), martial artist Artie Kaikou (who I have also known since my teens... he taught karate for years), Hawaiian fitness queen Dale Tomita (who went out of her way to be a complete diva the entire shoot and even complains a lot on film, you will see), masters body building champ Jesse Mathesen (who is seen bench pressing properly 405 for reps), Ms World Karen Hulse (who was the best of the bunch, taking over the filming on break without telling us, laughs), Ms Olympia Fitness Carol Semple (showing us her new braces for the first time in public) and Johnny Albert who runs the NPC Clothing Warehouse where we filmed again. It was a long day... We shot 12 noon to 12 midnight. "We shoot til we finish or til we drop." Everyone was in great shape. We did much better this time around with the exception of one girl thinking she was better than the rest, another upset because I wasn't interested in her, and the problems over a stolen car at the convention the day before. If it weren't for Dale acting like she was forced to be there, she signed an agreement to be there after all, and no one twisted her arm, everything went as well as it could I suppose.

I think we only forgot or ran out of time to film a few items this time.... No worries... A week later we shot in the gym I was sharing offices with a physician back in Youngstown, Ohio. Just a week after filming this third video, I have to admit, I was a little burnt out. The work, the stress, the divas... Ok, more than a little burnt out on divas...

What happened? I took the entire cast out for drinks and dancing the night afterwards only to have one of the girls get upset that I wasn't paying attention to her and didn't know how to treat a lady (I didn't see one). She got 'even' by telling everyone, while I was in the restroom, that I had left the club with someone else.... Not true... However, her plan to abandon me alone at the nightclub worked... I had to hitch a ride with some friends who luckily happened to be out the same evening...

What did I do about it once the weekend was over? Not much. Let's just say I wasn't the first to complain and her management dropped Miss Hessler shortly there after for related incidents... She of course claimed she wasn't compensated for her time but her management can attest that she was... Want to hear more about that? This is what management had to say:

DON LEMMON ASKED: What ever happened to some of the women I worked with in my videos? After Teresa Hessler pulled her stunt in Ohio at the one shoot, no matter how often I tell her it's alright, she won't face up to it all.

JM MANION OF JMP MANAGEMENT REPLIED: Whew. She was a problem in Ohio and everywhere else. I've held back on this for a couple of years, while she's told her side. This time, I am going to set the record straight. What it came down to was that she breached her contract with us numerous times. She accepted quite a few jobs behind our backs & didn't tell us. How I found out was I saw the print & video work she did. I don't know how she thought we'd never see this? At the time, she was living in the Baltimore area, then she met someone (behind her live-in boyfriend's back) & moved out to L.A. (only to fail there too)...

DON LEMMON ASKED: No way? Theresa? No..... But, but, she was so... Innocent.... Sweet... Honest...

JM MANION OF JMP MANAGEMENT REPLIED: Trust me, as I have the proof to back this up... So we consulted our attorney & set up terminating her contract, but not without getting our proper commission first. She immediately had a small mention in MuscleMag where she stated something to the effect that since she moved to California, JMP Management "couldn't" promote her any more. Anybody with any brains would know that Michelle Bellini lives in California & we were managing her at the time so why wouldn't we be able to manage Theresa? Carol Semple-Marzetta: Again, another athlete I've held back on discussing that breached her contract.

This third video features the ultra buff World Toughman Champ Ray Hammond (cool, cool guy) benching 500 pounds, Ms Fitness Ohio Michelle Talboo (and her daughter), Artie Kaikou who is shown teaching a martial arts class (where the kids undeservingly attack and beat me up, man, no respect) and Ms International Susie Curry training with me, rehearsing her fitness routine and even taking a Spinning class. The other video stars were model Brian Blazek (now a bartender at the Bellagio in Vegas, ladies), Theresa Hessler again and the always charming Danny Weigand. You might notice the bonus clips of Ms North America Ericca Kern but her footage was filmed a month later along with 2 other additional players. Ericca enjoys samples from our line of quintuple filtered, surgically pure, water in her closing shots. One thing in particular to note is that for the majority of our taping, the gyms were full of my real life clients hanging around, but let's ignore the toasts of wine we shared... Yes, I admit that's me having a beer with Pan Am games tae kwon do medallist Angela Wolbert and Susie Curry during a break!

The following day after the shoot, I took the group to hang out at the Mr Ohio Bodybuilding and Fitness show which I sponsored. I had a dozen people there and asked the video stars to hand out the trophies during the evening ceremony.

All in all, it really was a good time, maybe I just like to complain. Taking all of these larger than life people to my tiny little hometown of Newton Falls, Ohio or anywhere else all at once is simply asking for trouble. I cannot keep my eye on all of them and it adds up for problems no one could ever predict. The look on those little old ladies' faces when I came in with a bunch of comic book super heroes to my friend's small town diner was priceless. It was later that night the abandonment of yours truly occured...

Again, the CD of videos I am offering now are extremely educational but I can tell you that all day long and unless you have had experience with me in the past, you will believe it's just a sales pitch... I think you can tell, despite the things you learn, it's the antics you aren't expecting on an exercise or workout video that are worth the price of admission! In reality, all the problems on one shoot were due to the bad attitude of one girl spreading like poison to the rest of the cast and the same thing happening again with a different girl at fault on the next two shoots. If those three were eliminated, we probably would have went off without a single issue, besides editing.... None the less...

Definitely, if you listen to our discussions throughout the clips you will know the info couldn't be bought from any other trainer on earth. It's the drama, the headache, the senseless behavior... That's what I can't forget... The unnecessary delays during the editing process... Inexcusable holdups on top of uncooperative talent... Footage that either couldn't be used as planned or video that wasn't ready on time... Damaged goods... Combine it all together and a year after it all began, the summer of 1997... I sat with a letter in my hand stating the TV shopping channel that was once gung ho was no longer interested in my bringing my larger than life fitness stars to their airwaves. "Thank you people for your participation," they told me... No, thank YOU...
I lost money, investors lost money, I lost interest, I built a website...

And because of the success that this website has generated... I have had a change of heart... I am releasing what I have...

Since then, so much has changed. I am not implying my advice has changed but the methods I wish to promote or release it has. That's why, here we are, years later, after a long battle over rights, concepts and such, I have finally decided to release my exercise videos originally shot for QVC (one of the many American home shopping networks).

I know I just ranted for the past hour about how much my life sucked from June of 1996 to June of 1997 but truth be told, I am finally letting the public benefit from this work for the first time since it was completed and benefit you will by watching these videos.

Why is it in RAW Unedited format instead of completed, super high quality, over the top, ready for TV sort of stuff? As stated, the original editing was never completed as I requested. The original footage wasn't shot as I requested. While it may be 'alright' in the eyes of some people, I just couldn't accept things like speeding up a soundtrack to fit in shorter film segments, using angles not beneficial to the viewer... Oh, you get the point... And I was double charged for what was 'completed' leaving me little interest in redoing it all one more time. To top it off, after 6 years, I negotiated to buy the original tapes that the editor held while asking to get paid more than I initially agreed... And when they arrived... They wouldn't play! We tried everything, my wife is an expert on video production, and they were useless. Possibly stored next to something magnetic, but the footage... Lost... Forever... Except for the original dubs I was sent to review when we first shot it all...

And that is why we offering it RAW, unedited. Actually, I think this makes it much more charismatic. All the embarrassing parts are still intact, and so are the... You'll see...

ORDER A COPY OF ALL SIX HOURS, ALL 24 WORKOUTS, ALL 24 STARS, WELL OVER 100 EXERCISES AND STRETCHES, ALL ON ONE CD.... FOR ONLY $24.00! That is only ONE DOLLAR A WORKOUT! AND SHIPPING IS FREE IN THE USA!

Send your check or money order for $24.00 U.S. to us at:

Don Lemmon
590 Farrington Hwy 524-123
Kapolei, HI 96707

We accept only check or money order as this is a LIMITED TIME OFFER... If you do not order through this book you will notice that we will be doubled the price using your credit cards at the website... So why pay double when you can have it now for half price... And AUTOGRAPHED too? Also available at the same address are:

The 90 Day KNOW HOW Exercise & Menu Log PDF. If you want to detail your lifestyle and be 100% certain of why you succeed, why you are not succeeding and what really works... This is the book for you... It is a download, 8.5 x 11 inch pages and is available for a limited time for only $19.95 with FREE shipping!

KNOW HOW BOOK TWO... Another 300 pages full of NEW menus, workouts, recipes and extensive chapters exposing the personal training and body building industry by teaching you their secrets so you are no longer dependent. It's only $29.95 instead of $49.95 through the website! Why pay more?

This book teaches martial arts, bodybuilding, aerobics, boot camps, contest preparation, alternative health care, where to get free studies on everything your trainer and physician do not want you to online and more KNOW HOW that we all seek to own!

BONUS TWO! THE BEST BET IN GETTING STARTED!

I want you to try this for a while (and only these foods at these meals, change them only by telling me first as to not make mistakes, if you are a vegetarian, select only low carb alternatives to replace meats). Report back once you write up your first day's meal plan:

Breakfast upon awakening - have 1 'Perfect Vitamin' or a vitamin/mineral capsule, natural cereal, nonfat milk and fresh fruit, if you do not have the vitamins yet, take whatever is handy, same with herbs and glandulars, I take 3 Ultimate Herbal capsules per carb meal, do not worry if you do not have them yet….

Mid morning, 3 hours later or halfway between lunch and breakfast, snack - have 1 'Perfect Vitamin' or a vitamin/mineral capsule, 1 or 2 Glandular Complex capsules, nonfat cottage cheese (like it or not, start with a tablespoon one day, 2 the next, you'll grow on it) and Lemmon's oil, if you do not have the oil use unsweetened, unsalted almonds or nuts….

Lunch - have 1 'Perfect Vitamin' or a vitamin/mineral capsule, 1 or 2 Glandular Complex capsules, chicken, broccoli and a little butter (not margarine), taking several vitamins a day ensures you actually get any from the cheap products sold at stores, with ours, the amounts are broken down so you get 1/6 of what you need each serving…

Mid day, 3 hours later or halfway between lunch and dinner, snack - have 1 'Perfect Vitamin' or a vitamin/mineral capsule, 3 Ultimate Herb capsules, rice, beans and salsa, no oil, butter, or margarine…

Dinner - have 1 'Perfect Vitamin' or a vitamin/mineral capsule, 1 or 2 Glandular Complex capsules, red meat, a green salad and Lemmon's oil…

Mid evening, half way between bed and dinner, snack - have 1 'Perfect Vitamin' or a vitamin/mineral capsule, 1 or 2 Glandular Complex capsules, scrambled eggs and mushrooms, I suggest 2 whites for every 1 yolk by the way

- Variety of food comes down the road, do this now and in a few days we can make change, but you can't eat the same foods forever anymore than you can get started today worrying about it, let's go!
- Drink at least 24 ounces of water AFTER each feeding without fail but not with the meal...
- Eat as soon as you wake up each day, we know you do not exercise the second you wake nor do you need to delay the food so get rolling the second your eyes open and do not skip feedings during the day, pack your meals...
- Make sure each meal contains an equal amount of calories, not less at one, more at another, eat the same calories every feeding and READ LABELS...
- This is not a high fat diet and it is not all protein, low carb, nor is counting overall carbs/fats/protein ratios and percentages important....
- Keep the protein intake higher than fat but do not worry about how much for now....

For exercise, pick one exercise you know per body part and go do one set with whatever weight you like and see exactly how many reps you can perform without stopping. Move slow, raise and lower the weight 4 seconds up, 4 seconds down, quit the set when you feel you must and then report back the results. If you do not know movements to select, look here: http://www.exerciseandnutritionthetruth.com/exercises.html

Set this all up and plan to email it to me daily. We cannot be sure that you are on track unless you do and you MUST keep a daily record of all you do. Send it to me just as I have it here and only in an email NOT AN ATTACHMENT or Word File, etc:

Dear Don, my diet today was....

Meal 1 -
Meal 2 -
Meal 3 -
Meal 4 -
Meal 5 -
Meal 6 -

I want to know the foods and the times you ate the foods, etc. Next, send me your workout results:

Exercise 1 - Weight Used, Reps Performed
Exercise 2 - Weight Used, Reps Performed
Exercise 3 - Weight Used, Reps Performed

Etc for up to 10 exercises total and let me know how long the session was. Follow it up with cardio exercise, not before, but after the weights... Stretching too, which you will learn from my videos... What would I do if I was near a gym? When I workout at a club I do the following:

Chest machine presses
Military machine presses
Dips on parallel bars
Seated rowing machine
Underhand grip pulldowns
Bicep machine curls
Leg extensions
Leg curls
Leg presses

MAYBE.... I might do an abdominal exercise... Then I ride the bike or jog for 15 minutes MAXIMUM.

If you are on your feet most of the day, this is suffice for anyone.

If you are completely inactive, this is more than enough as you haven't been doing anything to begin with. If you feel you need more training, you aren't trying hard enough with the work you set out for yourself… You will see what I mean as we progress.

Do I really expect all people to have time for 6 to 7 feedings and still sleep? Lets see, here is the schedule of one client who emailed this week:

He wakes at 5 am…
Without hesitation, exercises til 5:30 a.m., then eats…
Next, he showers, drives to work, eats at 7:30 a.m. on the way…
Works until his first break at 10:30, eats again…
Lunch, 12:30 p.m., if unable to go to the cafeteria, has a Complete Protein Powder drink with Lemmon's Oil…
Mid day break 2:30 p.m., eats…
At 4:30 p.m. on the way home, eats lite so dinner isn't ruined…
6:00 p.m. is dinner…
8:00 p.m. is paperwork and a snack…
9:00 p.m. rolls around and it is time for bed…
….and this client is a surgeon…

Another is a foreman at an assembly factory and he has been eating when he wakes, during his first work break, lunch, mid day break, after work, dinner at home and a snack mid evening too... That's 7 again by the way.... And he has been fitting it in since he worked on the line 10 years ago.... So yes... Eat often. Even students have snacks between classes… So can you…

And please, comply with the above and I look forward to working together. The program starts NOW. Do what I recommend, forget what you think you know and the results will astound you whether you agree or understand…. In a week or so you will see what you have been missing. I appreciate you not only keeping this file private and to yourself because you paid for it, but this is how I earn my living. I thank you again.

WHAT MY CLIENTS HAVE TO SAY…

You may think my clients were all Los Angeles, California bodybuilders or models because of the folk you have seen endorsing or representing my videos, my web site or this book, but they weren't. Nearly a third of them yes, were from California, but another third were from Ohio and the final third came from Las Vegas, NV (not to mention all the people I have worked with on the internet).

These are the three major geographical areas where I have spent the majority of my life. Every one of them wanted the same things. To look better. To feel better. To do it easily. To never revert back to their old selves. Their age groups? From teenagers to centurions. High school students and senior citizens. Who did I like working with the most? Definitely I especially enjoyed the seniors. Life is so funny. We start off curious. We get to a point where we think we know it all. We progress past that to actually believing we really do know it all. Then we begin to worry about what we do not know and somewhere in the later years, we finally come to relax about knowing some things that just do not matter.

I will never say to myself 'if I knew then, what I know now' because that's not as important as making the proper decisions with what we have to base them on and then doing something to follow through with it all. The testimonials I receive regarding the success of my program are by far one of the more popular sections of my website. I can see why. Sometimes I look at them myself and forget people are writing about ME. Check it out sometime. It will be motivating to discover people you emulate are using the KNOW HOW. Actually, some of the people posted on my site were so appreciative of what the program did for them that they let me record phone interviews so we could make copies available to the public and we used to send them out for free in our supplement club packages. Everyone you meet in life will have radically different views.

These views stemming from their own personal experiences and backgrounds despite seeming so similar on the surface. Drop by the site and see if we have made these tapes available again or not. That's about all you will need to know in order to go into this system and have the program work for you too. The following pages contain statements made about the KNOW HOW system from people who substantiate the fact. You can not only learn from those who have triumphed from their decisions but also from other people's mistakes.

I think you'll be surprised by who's using The KNOW HOW system (not to mention where some of them have gotten using it). Thought those other programs are endorsed by the best? Guess again! I really can't think of a single program that can boast what I can.

Nonetheless, look who we have here today. Enjoy....

Kathy Faix, accountant, Youngstown, OH - "I've lost so many inches I'm almost embarrassed to discuss it! I've dropped a tremendous amount of fat and toned up REAL nice... Ask my husband Bob!" (She's lost 60 pounds of fat, gained 20 pounds of muscle in 6 months!)

Mark Mortimer, actor, New York, NY - "I do not trust anyone other than Don Lemmon with my exercise and nutrition recommendations. When I first got on his diet, I was able to improve my appearance on what is considered by most people to be a sorry excuse of a workout schedule and eating way too much food. I could not believe how much of a difference separating foods and exercising only twice a week has made!"

Kristi Davis, masseuse, Burbank, CA - "Finally! I feel comfortable about the way I look in clothes, when I go out, and in the mirror after getting out of the shower! And I feel tough too! Nothing like having strength! Girl Power!'

Larry Wolf, contractor, Hubbard, OH - "I was over 300 pounds and literally carrying 100 pounds of excess fat when I met Don. When he told me I could eat what ever I wanted, I said 'Great!' Since he taught me how to basically separate some foods from others and while doing just that, now eating whatever I want, no catches, I've lost 80 pounds of fat. The strange this is, I am eating more than ever!"

Michelle Ralabate, fitness model, Miami, FL - "This is a program worth endorsing! I think it is great that Don is telling it like it is for a change! When he asked me then to be one of his primary spokeswomen for 1996 I immediately said HECK YEAH! This guy has done a lot to help those in this industry who wanted to reach their goals without drugs."

Tony Fabrizzio, real estate agent, Las Vegas, NV - "Don's program works. I entered a natural (drug free) bodybuilding contest in 1995 promoted by Denny Kakos and even though the judges said I was listed on score cards as the winner, I was asked to withdraw at the last minute. The competitors protested saying nobody could look as ripped (lean) as I did without taking drugs! Well, I tested drug free and I was drug free."

Dr. Jean Williams, professor, Youngstown, OH - "I'm 65 and since meeting Mr. Lemmon I have been eating three times the food I normally would, lost over thirty pounds of fat and my doctor has taken me off medication that I've been on for over 30 years as a diabetic with lupus. Don is tough, but I have made more progress in the 3 months separating foods than I have with all other trainers and programs combined! Plus, my stomach pains are gone. That alone was worth the effort!"

Kiko Ellsworth, actor, Studio City, CA - "I got The KNOW HOW and after a couple weeks I am toppling my previous strength records and can already see my abs. It works well enough I just shot my own calendar."

Grace Grimes, fitness model, Cincinnati, OH - "I was brought up on hours of training sessions like everyone else. Don really knows his stuff though. I am living proof that proper nutrition and consistent exercise are the keys to success, weight loss, and even maintaining yourself! This program works for post pregnancy too by the way!"

Kevin Pugh, chef, Detroit, MI - "I personally didn't think it were possible, but this is an eating plan that not only works but fits into an everyday lifestyle. I have personally lost over 80 pounds in just four months. I've known Don for ten years and I waited much too long to do this."

Heather Pariso, Ms Internet World, Dover, OH - "I not only do not worry about fat sneaking up on me, but if it did this is the obvious logical approach to losing it! It is nice to know I can now get away with exercising so little and yet eating so much."

Dr. Dave Williams, chiropractor, Las Vegas, NV - "I have never read a book that surprised me like this one. I feel Don has put together something the entire World needs to see. He has worked with my Bishop, a surgeon friend, my lawyer and all our families. I recommend Don Lemmon and his theories to anyone and everyone. Our 6:30 a.m. workouts are good times I will never forget."

Marjean Holden, Beastmaster actress, New Zealand - "I'm really amazed at what my scale has told me! After losing several inches of blubber, I weigh the same as I did when I started but I look totally different! That must be muscle I gained while dropping fat right? Not bad."

Morris Sullivan, film producer, Toluca Lake, CA - "I was insulted at how simple the plan is. My strength at age 76 has never been better. I have gained 10 pounds of muscle though it looks like more and I am not even trying to lose fat but I am. Not bad for an old man. And my blood tests show a much younger man!"

Kelly Boling, secretary, Washington, DC - "I feel absolutely terrific. But even better than that, my mental acuity has improved tremendously. I swear I woke up this morning a dress size smaller too. My pants are fitting loosely, my stomach's flatter, my arms and legs look leaner, all in a month."

Dr. Robert Zeravica, chiropractor, Los Angeles, CA - "I honestly agree with every thing in this book. With so many nutritional programs on the market, I am amazed at how Don compiled all of this. Don's work should be required reading for all health care providers."

Laurie Donnelly, Ms Fitness America, Boulder, CO - "Don Lemmon certainly knows what he is doing! I was on a program similar to, but then again, nothing like Don's for my first year on television, which worked wonders. I and my two workout partners are giving Don a try without a bit of hesitation."

Artie Kaikou, martial artist, Akron, OH - "At first I didn't think it made sense but now it makes so much sense. I would have never achieved what I have without this KNOW HOW system. I tried for 10 years to get where I was able to get in just 10 weeks. I was 40 pounds lighter 3 months ago and I honestly feel I am not done yet. I can achieve anything now!"

Grace DeLaRosa, newscaster, The Big Island, HI - "There is nothing like knowing that you look good and have your health all year long. Too many times in the past I didn't want to do a shoot because I wasn't feeling my best. I guess you could say being on the Know How is like having extra money in your pocket!"

Brian Blazek, bartender, Henderson, NV - "I have added over 50 pounds to my bench, squat and dead lifts, 60 to my rows and gone from 45 to 65 pounds on my curls. Is this really possible? To top it all off, I seem to be literally repelling body fat as I get leaner and leaner by the moment!"

GET THE KNOW HOW ON AUDIO CD

Don Lemmon had been publishing books and marketing nutritional supplements for years and will not stand for his customers and readers to remain out of shape. The initial 5 times every 2 week weight lifting program is simple. If you've spent any time in the gym, you will be locked into the new routines in no time. But Lemmon also includes high-intensity tips to compound the training effect for more advanced clients. The same goes for the cardiovascular exercise he performs: just 12 minutes a session, five times every two week. But those 12 minutes are spent trying to accomplish more in less time. You have read about it all, now you can HEAR about it all and finally, truly grasp all the nutritional, exercise and motivational tips.

Don Lemmon is many things to the people who listen to this audiotape: personal trainer, motivational guru, nutrition consultant, lifestyle and success coach. As you listen to Alan Blair read Don's best selling internet book, he inspires, excites, instructs, and sometimes gives listeners something they aren't expecting... An end to making excuses.

The goal is for the listener to transform his or her body and in the process learn that changing your outsides also changes the insides. This audio book is something the fans have been asking for since 1996. Just mention the name Don Lemmon to any of the people he's helped and you will see their respect in their eyes. You will hear it in their words. These people include thousands of men and women who sought out for help and found straight forward advice they could live with. And now, for the first time ever... You can keep motivated by listening to Don Lemmon's work whenever you need to... And by ordering through us... SHIPPING IS FREE IN THE USA!

Send your check or money order for $30.00 U.S. to:

Don Lemmon, 590 Farrington Hwy 524-123, Kapolei, HI 96707

DON LEMMON'S NUTRITION, MENU & DIET SOFTWARE

Don Lemmon's Know How Nutritional Software is simple to use and will prove to be very helpful in achieving your nutritional goals. You download the software to your computer from the CD and it opens in literally seconds.

Next, you select your height, weight, waist measure, and your current body weight. Selecting whether you were male or female follows. This info gives the program an idea of what your body fat levels have.

And this is crucial info. Everyone's height has a specific waist measure. Knowing how far off you are allows the system to dictate whether you need to gain, lose or maintain your current condition.

If you know them (not required) you can either put in the grams or calories of what you eaten on the average per day for the past week straight.

That's proteins, carbohydrates and fats if possible. Or just calories... And that's it. You are practically done!

From there it gives you a specific set of meals to follow, suiting your goal to take you from where you are now and covers the next 30 days of your life. In fact, you get over a dozen menu plans during the month long plan.

You get exact calories you'll need to succeed or reach your goals; the software has the ability to print out the menu information and it's as simple as a click of a button; it also includes a complete shopping list... And this entire process happens all within 1 or 2 minutes from your initial download.

It begins calculating every time you enter new info too.... Lickety SPLIT! BAM! Enter in a family member... DONE!

It's that EASY! That's all the more thinking it takes, so no more guess work in how much to eat or what prepare any longer!

We have actually made it so you can succeed without even reading the Don Lemmon's nutrition and exercise book and that goes for even if you are on another program!

How so? It doesn't matter if you are on a low carbohydrates, low fat, balanced macro nutrient or vegetarian menu.... Just insert your info and print out the diets. You will be taken from where you are now and put completely on track for what works over the next 30 days...

Amazing huh? No one does this. All diets are modified using the Don Lemmon philosophy to allow for optimal digestion, health and progress...

What if you did not like a particular food on these diets? Again... No problem! That is what our FREE ONLINE COUNSELING IS FOR!

What does all of this mean? It means you have no more limitations. Sometimes certain questions just can't be answered by a book, no matter how hard we try to cover all the bases.

I understand this and that is why I allow you to contact me with your questions online, schedule personal phone calls or even consultations in my office.

To order Don Lemmon's software, SHIPPING IS FREE IN THE USA! Send your check or money order for $20.00 U.S. to:

Don Lemmon 590 Farrington Hwy 524-123 Kapolei, HI 96707

FOR OUR SPECIALS, OTHER THREE BOOKS, ETC.
www.ExerciseAndNutritionTheTruth.com